COPING WITH TH

CAROLINE CLAYTON is a jou
interest in women's health. She first wrote about the problems of thrush in *Company* magazine. The response from sufferers prompted her to write this book, to offer them help and information. Caroline is the author of *Coping with Cystitis*, also published by Sheldon Press.

Overcoming Common Problems Series

For a full list of titles please contact
Sheldon Press, Marylebone Road, London NW1 4DU

Antioxidants
DR ROBERT YOUNGSON

The Assertiveness Workbook
A plan for busy women
JOANNA GUTMANN

Beating the Comfort Trap
DR WINDY DRYDEN AND JACK GORDON

Birth Over Thirty Five
SHEILA KITZINGER

Body Language
How to read others' thoughts by their gestures
ALLAN PEASE

Body Language in Relationships
DAVID COHEN

Calm Down
How to cope with frustration and anger
DR PAUL HAUCK

Cancer – A Family Affair
NEVILLE SHONE

The Cancer Guide for Men
HELEN BEARE AND NEIL PRIDDY

The Candida Diet Book
KAREN BRODY

Caring for Your Elderly Parent
JULIA BURTON-JONES

Cider Vinegar
MARGARET HILLS

Comfort for Depression
JANET HORWOOD

Coping Successfully with Hayfever
DR ROBERT YOUNGSON

Coping Successfully with Joint Replacement
DR TOM SMITH

Coping Successfully with Migraine
SUE DYSON

Coping Successfully with Pain
NEVILLE SHONE

Coping Successfully with Panic Attacks
SHIRLEY TRICKETT

Coping Successfully with PMS
KAREN EVENNETT

Coping Successfully with Prostate Problems
ROSY REYNOLDS

Coping Successfully with Your Hiatus Hernia
DR TOM SMITH

Coping Successfully with Your Irritable Bladder
JENNIFER HUNT

Coping Successfully with Your Irritable Bowel
ROSEMARY NICOL

Coping with Anxiety and Depression
SHIRLEY TRICKETT

Coping with Blushing
DR ROBERT EDELMANN

Coping with Breast Cancer
DR EADIE HEYDERMAN

Coping with Bronchitis and Emphysema
DR TOM SMITH

Coping with Candida
SHIRLEY TRICKETT

Coping with Chronic Fatigue
TRUDIE CHALDER

Coping with Coeliac Disease
KAREN BRODY

Coping with Cystitis
CAROLINE CLAYTON

Coping with Depression and Elation
DR PATRICK McKEON

Coping with Eczema
DR ROBERT YOUNGSON

Coping with Endometriosis
JO MEARS

Coping with Fibroids
MARY-CLAIRE MASON

Coping with Headaches
SHIRLEY TRICKETT

Coping with a Hernia
DR DAVID DELVIN

Coping with Psoriasis
PROFESSOR RONALD MARKS

Coping with Rheumatism and Arthritis
DR ROBERT YOUNGSON

Coping with Stammering
TRUDY STEWART AND JACKIE TURNBULL

Coping with Stomach Ulcers
DR TOM SMITH

Overcoming Common Problems Series

Coping with Strokes
DR TOM SMITH

Coping with Thrush
CAROLINE CLAYTON

Coping with Thyroid Problems
DR JOAN GOMEZ

Coping with Your Cervical Smear
KAREN EVENNETT

Crunch Points for Couples
JULIA COLE

Curing Arthritis
More ways to a drug-free life
MARGARET HILLS

Curing Arthritis Diet Book
MARGARET HILLS

Curing Arthritis – The Drug-Free Way
MARGARET HILLS

Curing Arthritis Exercise Book
MARGARET HILLS AND JANET HORWOOD

Cystic Fibrosis – A Family Affair
JANE CHUMBLEY

Depression
DR PAUL HAUCK

Divorce and Separation
Every woman's guide to a new life
ANGELA WILLANS

Everything Parents Should Know About Drugs
SARAH LAWSON

Feverfew
DR STEWART JOHNSON

Gambling – A Family Affair
ANGELA WILLANS

Garlic
KAREN EVENNETT

The Good Stress Guide
MARY HARTLEY

Heart Attacks – Prevent and Survive
DR TOM SMITH

Helping Children Cope with Attention Deficit Disorder
DR PATRICIA GILBERT

Helping Children Cope with Bullying
SARAH LAWSON

Helping Children Cope with Divorce
ROSEMARY WELLS

Helping Children Cope with Dyslexia
SALLY RAYMOND

Helping Children Cope with Grief
ROSEMARY WELLS

Helping Children Cope with Stammering
JACKIE TURNBULL AND TRUDY STEWART

Hold Your Head Up High
DR PAUL HAUCK

How to Be Your Own Best Friend
DR PAUL HAUCK

How to Cope When the Going Gets Tough
DR WINDY DRYDEN AND JACK GORDON

How to Cope with Anaemia
DR JOAN GOMEZ

How to Cope with Bulimia
DR JOAN GOMEZ

How to Cope with Difficult Parents
DR WINDY DRYDEN AND JACK GORDON

How to Cope with Difficult People
ALAN HOUEL WITH CHRISTIAN GODEFROY

How to Cope with People who Drive You Crazy
DR PAUL HAUCK

How to Cope with Splitting Up
VERA PEIFFER

How to Cope with Stress
DR PETER TYRER

How to Enjoy Your Retirement
VICKY MAUD

How to Improve Your Confidence
DR KENNETH HAMBLY

How to Interview and Be Interviewed
MICHELE BROWN AND GYLES BRANDRETH

How to Keep Your Cholesterol in Check
DR ROBERT POVEY

How to Love and Be Loved
DR PAUL HAUCK

How to Pass Your Driving Test
DONALD RIDLAND

How to Stand up for Yourself
DR PAUL HAUCK

How to Start a Conversation and Make Friends
DON GABOR

How to Stick to a Diet
DEBORAH STEINBERG AND DR WINDY DRYDEN

How to Stop Worrying
DR FRANK TALLIS

Overcoming Common Problems Series

How to Succeed as a Single Parent
CAROLE BALDOCK

How to Untangle Your Emotional Knots
DR WINDY DRYDEN AND JACK GORDON

How to Write a Successful CV
JOANNA GUTMANN

Hysterectomy
SUZIE HAYMAN

The Incredible Sulk
DR WINDY DRYDEN

The Irritable Bowel Diet Book
ROSEMARY NICOL

The Irritable Bowel Stress Book
ROSEMARY NICOL

Is HRT Right for You?
DR ANNE MACGREGOR

Jealousy
DR PAUL HAUCK

Learning to Live with Multiple Sclerosis
DR ROBERT POVEY, ROBIN DOWIE AND GILLIAN PRETT

Living with Angina
DR TOM SMITH

Living with Asthma
DR ROBERT YOUNGSON

Living with Diabetes
DR JOAN GOMEZ

Living with Grief
DR TONY LAKE

Living with High Blood Pressure
DR TOM SMITH

Living with a Stoma
DR CRAIG WHITE

Making the Most of Yourself
GILL FOX AND SHEILA DAINOW

Menopause
RAEWYN MACKENZIE

The Migraine Diet Book
SUE DYSON

Motor Neurone Disease – A Family Affair
DR DAVID OLIVER

The Nervous Person's Companion
DR KENNETH HAMBLY

Out of Work – A Family Affair
ANNE LOVELL

Overcoming Anger
DR WINDY DRYDEN

Overcoming Guilt
DR WINDY DRYDEN

Overcoming Jealousy
DR WINDY DRYDEN

Overcoming Shame
DR WINDY DRYDEN

The Parkinson's Disease Handbook
DR RICHARD GODWIN-AUSTEN

The PMS Diet Book
KAREN EVENNETT

A Positive Thought for Every Day
DR WINDY DRYDEN

Second Time Around
ANNE LOVELL

Serious Mental Illness – A Family Affair
GWEN HOWE

Sex and Relationships
ROSEMARY STONES

The Stress Workbook
JOANNA GUTMANN

The Subfertility Handbook
VIRGINIA IRONSIDE AND SARAH BIGGS

Talking About Anorexia
How to cope with life without starving
MAROUSHKA MONRO

Talking with Confidence
DON GABOR

Ten Steps to Positive Living
DR WINDY DRYDEN

Think Your Way to Happiness
DR WINDY DRYDEN AND JACK GORDON

Understanding Obsessions and Compulsions
A self-help manual
DR FRANK TALLIS

Understanding Your Personality
Myers-Briggs and more
PATRICIA HEDGES

Overcoming Common Problems

COPING WITH THRUSH

Caroline Clayton

sheldon PRESS

First published in Great Britain in 1984 by
Sheldon Press, SPCK, Marylebone Road, London NW1 4DU
as **Thrush: How it's caused and what to do about it**

Revised, updated edition 1994
Fourth impression 2001

British Library Cataloguing-in-Publication Data

A catalogue record for this book is available from the British Library

ISBN 0–85969–697–9

Photoset by Deltatype Ltd, Birkenhead, Merseyside
Printed in Great Britain by Biddles Ltd, *www.biddles.co.uk*

Contents

To Mike and Max

Acknowledgements

I would like to express my sincerest gratitude to the following people for supplying information so promptly, together with kind advice and assistance: Professor Michael Adler, Dr J. M. Emens, Dr Hilary Tillett, Dr E. Wilson-Kay, David Mitchell at Janssen Pharmacy Division, Nicola Wilcox at Bayer PLC, Jennifer Adams at Pfizer Limited, The House of Mistry, Sharon Clark at the London Rubber Company, the Health Education Authority, Joe Tallantire and the Women's Environmental Network, The Women's Health Information Centre, Judith Brett, Karena Callen, Mike Clowes, Jacqui Deevoy, Sally Dickens, Shelley Gare and Maggie Goodman, Caroline Harper, Tracey King, Andrea Pinnington, and Sally Ruth (my friend in New Zealand).

I would also like to thank all the women who wrote to me and gave me so much encouragement and support. This book is for them.

Introduction

Every year millions of women get vaginal thrush. Nearly three out of four women will have at least one attack during their lifetime, and many will get it more than once.

Second only to cystitis, thrush causes more misery for more women than any other minor illness. Indeed, thrush is a most distressing and depressing condition, especially when it recurs. Thrush affects us physiologically and psychologically. It affects our attitudes to our bodies.

Many women find it hard to talk about vaginal infections, but, if you suffer from thrush, you will need to know more about it to help you cope. Thrush *can* be cured — if not with drugs, then with simple, easy-to-use home remedies. And thrush can be *prevented*.

This is a self-help book. It explains why we get thrush, how we can get rid of it when we have got it, and how we can avoid getting it again. It will teach you how to recognize the symptoms of thrush and how not to confuse them with other more serious infections. It will advise you how to treat yourself or tell you where to go to get help. More importantly, it describes many ways in which you can help yourself.

This book also aims to put a new perspective on recurrent thrush. Recurrent thrush occurs for a very simple reason, but, in the past, many sufferers have been told that 'they must learn to live with it' or, to put it bluntly, to 'put up and shut up'!

I hope that this book will show anyone concerned about thrush that there *is* an alternative; there is no reason to suffer any more.

1
What is thrush?

I didn't even realize I had thrush for a while. I had a white discharge, but it wasn't smelly and only slightly heavier than normal.

I was in agony. My vagina was sore and red and I had a very heavy, thick, curdy discharge.

When I got thrush I knew something was wrong straight away. I was so sore and swollen 'down there' I could hardly walk!

It was very painful having sex.

I couldn't stop itching myself. I scratched myself in my sleep and made myself bleed!

These are the words of women describing what it feels like when you have thrush. The symptoms they describe are generally recognized as signs of thrush, although not everyone with the infection will suffer from the full range of symptoms, as you can see. What exactly is thrush, though, and where does it come from?

Thrush is a fungal infection, rather like athlete's foot, and it is caused by the yeast-like organism, *Candida albicans*. Although the medical name for thrush is *Candida*, it may also be called *Moniliasis*, yeast infection, the whites or fungus. It does not come from anywhere. *Candida* is naturally present in the vagina and bowel, along with a multitude of other different bacteria and fungi. The acidity of the vagina prevents yeasts and other potentially harmful organisms from multiplying out of all proportion. It is only when the delicate pH balance (acid/alkaline) of the vagina is upset that the 'threatening' bacteria take hold and infections occur.

The warmth and moisture of the vagina provides an ideal environment for the fungus to grow. It is also possible, however, to get thrush in the mouth, intestine or bowel and, in some cases, even in the lungs. In fact, it thrives anywhere that is damp and wet. The fungus multiplies rapidly, but, like all yeast, it feeds on and needs sugar to grow, which is why diet plays such an important part in the treatment of thrush. It does not always produce a discharge but is usually very itchy, and makes the whole of the genital area inflamed and sore.

Most cases of thrush arise spontaneously. This really means that they come about because of certain changes that have occurred within the body. Thrush is not necessarily caught from another person. Babies and little children can suffer with thrush just as much as adult men and women can. However, thrush is sexually transmissible. If you have thrush and you are sexually active, it is very important that your partner or partners are treated, too. It is also possible to carry thrush without knowing it as it may not give rise to any symptoms. This is why both partners must be treated for thrush even if only one of you is actually 'suffering'. Thrush may also be transferred by hand, so it is not confined to heterosexual relationships.

It is especially important to remember that every attack of thrush, whether it has been acquired sexually or not, can be passed on. More often than not, thrush is usually only 'carried' by the male sexual partner. In most, but not all cases, it does not give rise to symptoms. The male here will be a constant source of reinfection unless he, too, is treated. In men, thrush tends to manifest itself as a urinary infection. Doctors call it non-specific urethritis (NSU). This is an inflammation or infection of the urethra, the tube that carries urine from the bladder to the outside of the body. It makes you want to urinate frequently, although there may be little or no water to pass. Urinating is painful, causing a burning or stinging sensation. You may even begin to pass blood. NSU is becoming an increasing concern of doctors in uro-genital medicine. It is regarded as a far more serious complaint than thrush as, if left untreated, it can develop into Reiter's Disease. This is a form of arthritis, which can be crippling. The eyes may also be affected, and some men develop skin and mouth lesions. Like thrush, NSU is frequently recurrent. Women should not ignore NSU because, as carriers, they can reinfect their partner or partners. Men with NSU should always make sure that they are treated for thrush as well, if the attack is linked with it.

Recurrent thrush

Some days I get so depressed. The itching and irritation nearly drives me mad.

When I went to my doctor last month for a prescription, I was told I wouldn't have to put up with it all my life — I'd lose it when

> I got to the menopause. I told him I felt as if I'd had it all my life now. It's not a very comforting thought to think I might have to go like this for another ten years.
>
> Honestly, it's got to the stage where I don't feel like a woman any more.

Thrush as an infection, as we have seen, is not usually serious. But for those sufferers who cannot seem to shake it off and spend weeks, months and sometimes years with recurrent attacks, thrush can cause great emotional damage.

This book deals mainly with vaginal thrush because this is where, more often than not, the effects of thrush make themselves known to most women. Recurrent vaginal thrush is now thought to be a symptom that thrush is present throughout the body, so it really is a different problem to a one-off, isolated attack. A study by M. R. Miles, L. Olsen and A. Rogers ('Recurrent Vaginal Candidiasis: The importance of an intestinal reservoir' *JAMA*, 1977, 234, 1836) examined 98 women who complained of recurrent vaginal thrush. The results were amazing. Swabs were inserted into the vagina and bowel of each woman and compared with the results from the other women. It was found that thrush was *always* present in the bowel if it was found in the vagina. Those who tested negative for thrush in the bowel *never* showed positive for *Candida* in the vagina.

These findings would seem to prove that an excess of thrush in the vagina is simply a symptom of a general *Candida* problem that must be treated. Anyone who suffers from repeated attacks of thrush must be treated systematically. That means asking your doctor for an oral drug like Diflucan or Sporanox (see Chapter 5) and/or self-treating your system by eating lots of live yogurt and sticking to an anti-*Candida* diet (see Chapter 7) to clear the whole body of the problem.

Many women have resigned themselves to being recurrent thrush sufferers. This is totally unnecessary, as this book will show. However, it is important here to define what recurrent thrush *is*. There is a difference between one-off, uncomplicated doses of vaginal thrush occurring and attacks recurring so frequently that the sufferer seems to have permanent thrush. Two attacks in six months are probably unconnected. If you have three or more attacks in this short space of time, though, it is likely that you have an overall thrush infestation that needs treatment.

There is, however, another important explanation for recurrent thrush. It is possible that patients suffering from repeated attacks may be being reinfected by their sexual partner(s). This is why it is so important that sexually active sufferers get their partners checked out, too. Do not start having sex again until you have been given the 'all clear'. Women (and men) prone to thrush could try the condom as a method of contraception in future to minimize the chances of reinfection.

Complications of thrush

It is now believed that although thrush in itself is not a serious disease, left unchecked it can cause problems. A *Candida* overgrowth in the intestines can damage the mucus-covered lining here and lead to *leaky gut syndrome*. This is explained in more detail in Chapter 7, but, essentially, what happens is that, instead of being passed out of the body, as normally happens, harmful organisms in the bowel can become reabsorbed into the digestive system. This can cause headaches, dizziness, faintness, nausea and acne or food allergies to develop. Chronic *Candida* throughout the body may cause more serious conditions, such as asthma and psoriasis.

It has been suggested that women with thrush might be temporarily infertile when there is a lot of thrush around the neck of the womb, or cervix. If you have been trying unsuccessfully to conceive and have a recurrent thrush problem, it is possible to check whether thrush could be a cause of this.

Scientists have also drawn a link between thrush and premenstrual tension (PMT). A recent study looked at women suffering from both PMT and thrush. The survey discovered that two-thirds of the women's PMT improved when their thrush was treated with antifungal drugs and diet. PMT may just be a symptom of too much *Candida* in the body. So, PMT sufferers with a history of vaginal thrush will probably be helped by an anti-*Candida* programme.

Extreme cases of candidiasis have been linked with myalgic encephalomyelitis (ME). This is thought to be a viral condition, although some doctors do not recognize it as an illness. ME used to be called 'Yuppy Flu', mainly because the sufferers whose case histories were highlighted in the media tended to be high achievers with stressful lives. However, this classification was misleading as ME affects a broad range of people from all walks of life.

Interestingly, the symptoms ME sufferers complain of are also experienced by sufferers of chronic thrush — extreme fatigue, depression, lack of concentration and poor memory. Also, when given treatment for *Candida* through drugs and diet, ME sufferers' symptoms have often disappeared!

The best way to fight thrush is to treat your body as a whole. This book will show you how.

Oral thrush

As mentioned earlier, it is possible to get thrush in other parts of the body. Overweight people who have deep skin folds where sweat gathers are prone to *Candida* infections in such places. Young babies and the elderly seem particularly susceptible to thrush in the mouth, but infections here are easily diagnosed. White deposits will be noticeable on the tongue and around the insides of the mouth, and white plaques collect at its corners. Sufferers might also experience a sore or dry mouth, with a burning sensation that gets worse on eating. Denture wearers might notice that their gums become sore, red and inflamed.

Oral thrush is unusual in adults, unless they have just taken antibiotics or steroids. Anyone with an unexplained attack of thrush in the mouth should consult their doctor immediately.

There is more about oral thrush in Chapters 2 and 10. But remember, the best way to cure it is to prevent it occurring in the first place!

A women's problem

Thrush is mainly a women's problem, and to understand *why* women get thrush we need to know a little about the female sexual and reproductive organs. The diagrams on page 8 show these in detail.

The surface sex organs (the vulva) are protected by a pair of outer lips — the labia majora. The urethral and vaginal openings are enclosed within a second pair of lips — the labia minora. The area between these inner lips and the anus is called the perineum.

The close proximity of the anus, vagina and urethra helps to explain why women suffer so much with genital infections. Notice how near the urinary opening is to the vagina. Vaginal infections invariably work their way up to the urethra, and can lead to urinary

External sex organs

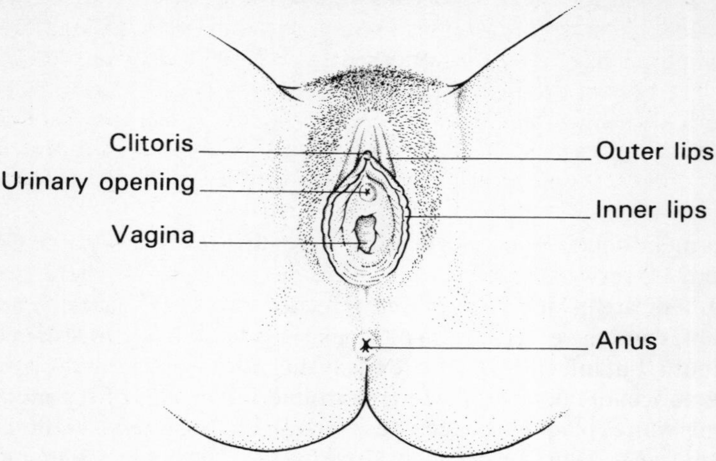

Internal sexual/reproductive organs

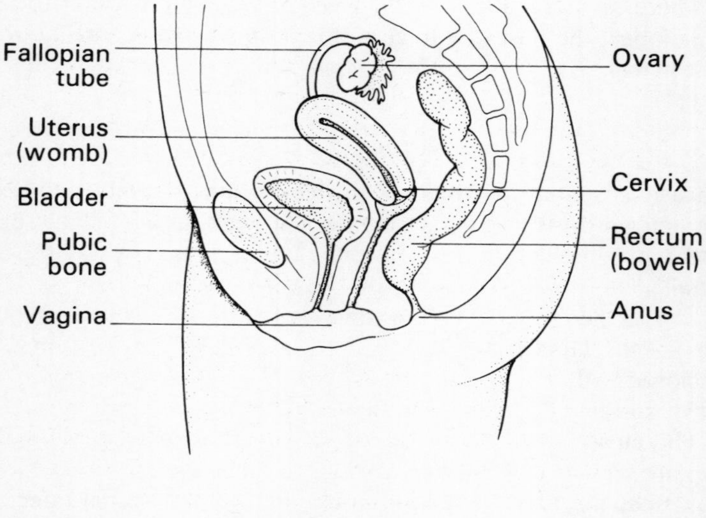

infections. Once the infection reaches the bladder, it will not be long before the kidneys are affected, too. Many infections, including thrush, arise because bacteria from the anus reach the vagina. Hygiene is vital to prevent germs spreading around the vulva. But, as you will see, cleanliness alone cannot protect you against thrush.

The vulva is full of tiny crevices and folds of skin – places where thrush loves to hide. Because of this, treatment that concentrates on the vagina alone is not always sufficient to clear up an attack. Women with thrush should ask for an antifungal cream (see Chapter 5) to smear around the labia to eradicate any fungi that might be lurking here.

So, not only does the female anatomy make women more susceptible to thrush, it also makes it harder to get rid of. Men are not so frequently afflicted with it, simply because they do not have a place like a vagina where the fungus can breed so well. When thrush does occur in a man, it will usually have been contracted sexually, and it flares up under the foreskin. This means that circumcized men have even less chance of getting thrush. Remember that it is just as much a man's responsibility to prevent the spread of infection where it can be helped as it is a woman's.

As a sufferer, you will get to know what thrush feels like so that you will probably realize when an attack is beginning. For most people, the first attack is the worst simply because they do not understand what is wrong. It is very tempting to scratch a furious itch or soak for several hours in a hot bath and hope that the trouble goes away. Taking this sort of action to relieve the symptoms, however, is misguided and ineffective as soaking in hot water can actually help *Candida* to multiply, by making the vagina warmer and wetter. Avoid scratching, which irritates and spreads infection.

The following are the warning signals of a vaginal infection:

- soreness or dryness (it is normal to have a wetness or secretion from the vagina)
- itching or burning
- rashes or sore spots on the genitals
- a strong-smelling or frothing discharge
- a dark-coloured discharge (vaginal moisture is normally clear or slightly milky)
- an urge to pass water a lot and pain when doing so.

If you notice any of these symptoms, get medical help immediately. The symptoms of thrush can sometimes be confused with other vaginal infections, which is why it is best to consult a doctor whenever you think you have thrush, and *essential* if you have any of the symptoms just mentioned. When one infection begins in the genital area, it is very easy for another to start up, too! On a final note, it must be stressed that when you are being treated for any infection, never stop taking the treatment just because the symptoms disappear; it is very important to take a *full* course of treatment for an effective and lasting cure.

2

How do you get it?

If you have never suffered from thrush before, you might be a little surprised to learn how common it is. Research has shown that seven out of ten women will have at least one attack during their lifetime, and many will get it more than once. Often, too, *Candida* is found in a patient even though they do not have any symptoms of the infection. It is thought that about a third of the Western population has a *Candida* problem.

Chapter 1 explained that women tend to suffer from thrush more often than men. We are more susceptible to the infection because a woman's vagina can offer the perfect breeding ground for thrush to take a hold, so let us now look at how this happens in more detail.

The vagina

Throughout our menstrual cycle, the vagina secretes its slippery fluids. It is perfectly normal for the walls of the vagina to feel wet — indeed, it is this moisture that helps to keep the vagina healthy, by keeping it clean and comfortable. The continuous secretion provides lubrication. Without it, sex would not only be less enjoyable but also less comfortable.

Vaginal moisture is clear or somewhat milky. It tastes slightly salty and dries to a faint whitish yellow colour. This may be noticeable on your underwear. The amount of wetness and its consistency varies throughout the menstrual cycle. It increases when we become sexually aroused. After the menopause, the vagina loses some of its moisture and elasticity. Usually this only occurs in the latter part of the menopause, about five to ten years after the last period. The lack of fluid can cause irritation so that during intercourse a substitute for the missing lubrication may be necessary.

A dry vagina is far more susceptible to infection. When the tender mucous membranes are inflamed and sore, infections find it easier to take a hold. This is why it is important not to have intercourse unless you are feeling sexually healthy. If penetration is difficult – and it will be if the vagina is dry or closed up – the delicate tissues are damaged. This makes the perineum sore, and makes a vaginal infection a hundred times worse.

The natural moisture of the vagina has yet another function. It helps maintain the acidity of the vagina and so prevents infections from starting. The mucus secreted by the walls of the vagina contains glycogen. This is a sugary substance. It is fermented into lactic acid by the normal bacteria (*lactobacilli*) in the vagina. Lactic acid is the same sort of acid as that formed in the making of yogurt, which inhibits fungal growth.

The PH scale

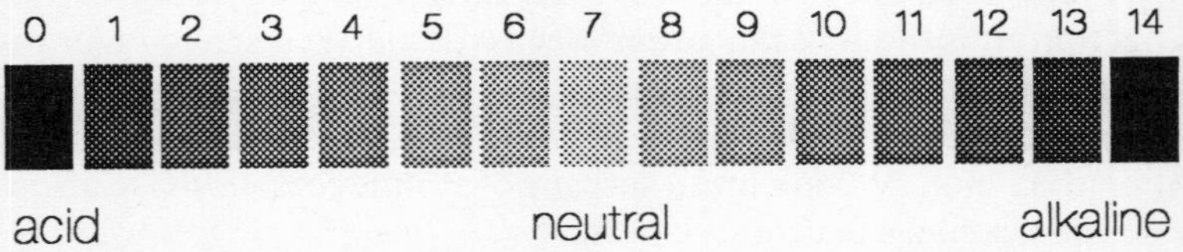

The natural pH balance of the vagina is usually somewhere around 4.0 to 5.0. During menstruation, the pH balance rises to 5.8 or 6.8 because blood is alkaline. As thrush and other infections thrive best in the least acidic conditions, you are more vulnerable at this time of the month than at any other.

There are a number of other changes that can take place within our bodies to alter the natural environment of the vagina. Anything that disturbs the flora, or ecological balance, of *lactobacilli* and other bacteria in the vagina will create conditions that allow thrush and other infections to flare up.

In summary, the vagina and sex organs are affected by the presence of *alkalinity*, and/or the *lack of protective bacteria*. Fungi multiply rapidly in warm, moist conditions so that *humidity* can disturb the vagina's ecology. Too much *sugar* can also cause problems — *Candida* needs sugar for growth. These are the main reasons why we get thrush. If you have a recurrent thrush problem, it may be because the infection has never been properly cleared, but is being constantly aggravated by one or more of these conditions. I shall now go on to examine the sort of things that may precipitate an attack of thrush, and which may have a harmful effect on the vagina.

The Pill

Women on the Pill are more likely to develop thrush than those using other forms of contraception. There are three types of oral contraceptive: combined oestrogen/progestogen preparations, sequential preparations containing oestrogens and progestogens, and the progestogen-only Pill. Oestrogen is one of the female sex hormones. The amount released into the body at any one time depends on what stage a woman is at in her menstrual cycle. It is this amount that helps to make the cycle work. The hormone is present in much higher levels during pregnancy. When you take an oestrogen-based oral contraceptive, this has the same effect on the body as pregnancy. It is quite usual for pregnant women to develop thrush. When you are pregnant, there is an increase in the glycogen content of the vaginal mucus. If too much glycogen (sugar) is produced and is not broken down into an acidic form, the vagina loses its natural protection against fungal infections. Pregnant women are thus more vulnerable to the growth of *Candida albicans* (see Chapter 10).

One of the ways in which the Pill works is by increasing the vagina's natural secretions. The thickening of the mucus in the cervical canal prevents sperm from entering the uterus. The additional moisture in and around the vagina can aggravate a recurrent thrush problem. The progestogen-only Pill works almost entirely on the principle that progestogen increases cervical mucus. The increased moisture can actually encourage the fungus to thrive! This type of Pill has another disadvantage. One of its side-effects is heavier and more frequent periods. Breakthrough bleeding (bleeding between periods) is not uncommon. These may also provoke vaginal thrush. For some women, especially those whose thrush tends to return with a period, prolonged bleeding would be a nightmare.

Cervical eversion

Another of the problems the Pill presents is that it can cause *cervical eversion*, which, in turn, can be a cause of thrush (see Chapter 9). An eversion (sometimes called an 'erosion') means that the soft, red cells from inside the cervix have grown outside it. The hormone oestrogen in the Pill brings this about. Again, this is a normal occurrence in pregnancy. When an eversion becomes infected — and it will, if you get an attack of thrush — the most effective treatment is to deal with the eversion itself. This can be done in one of two ways: by cauterizing, or burning off the layer of cells, or with cryosurgery, or freezing them off. These processes should only be carried out if the eversion becomes troublesome or if infections are recurrent. They are, therefore, valid in the case of recurrent thrush. Both treatments work very well, but they do not last forever. Cervical eversion, once it has happened, tends to continue. There is little use, therefore, in treating an eversion with cautery or cryosurgery if the oestrogen that caused it in the first place is not reduced. This may mean coming off the Pill.

The Pill is the most effective form of contraception we have to date. For many people it is *the* most effective contraception. Anyone who is considering changing from oral contraception to another sort should, of course, think the matter over very carefully. For those whose thrush is 'oestrogen orientated' switching to the progestogen-only Pill may do the trick and clear it up. The main drawback in using this particular Pill is that it is not as efficient in preventing pregnancy as the other available types of oral contraceptives. There is a much greater risk of pregnancy if you forget to take one of these Pills. If one is missed, the course should be continued as usual, but do not have sex on that particular day. Just to be on the safe side, an additional precaution, such as a condom, should be used until the next period.

> I only found out that the contraceptive pill aggravates thrush some six months ago. A specialist suggested that I abstain from taking the Pill for a short while. I did so and my condition improved. I went back on a different Pill at her suggestion. The thrush infection returned. I stopped the Pill altogether at my own discretion. In my case, the Pill itself was the sole cause of the thrush infection.

> I was taking the contraceptive pill for three years before it occurred, having nearly gone mad with itching for three days before I could get an appointment with my GP. TCP cream, I found, eased the irritation slightly, although the aroma wasn't too good.
>
> Anyway, my GP diagnosed my dilemma as thrush — stating that the Pill can aggravate the situation. He prescribed a course of six pessaries (Canesten) for three days' use. One week later, the thrush had returned with a vengeance, so back I went again to my GP, who prescribed a one-week course of Nystatin pessaries plus some cream. This luckily worked, but I decided to give up the Pill because of the hassle.

If you are thinking about changing your method of contraception, it is best to talk about it with your doctor or, better still, at a family planning clinic. They will discuss all the options open to you in birth control. The clinic will keep a constant check on your health through successive visits. If you do stop taking the Pill, remember that no other contraceptive will be so easy to use. The condom and the cap must be used properly if they are to be effective. This means using them every time and before sexual contact begins, whether or not both partners intend to continue making love until orgasm. The condom has one big advantage for thrush sufferers — it is a barrier method. It prevents full contact between sexual partners during intercourse, but it also prevents you reinfecting each other, and that cannot be bad!

Sometimes a short break from the Pill, perhaps for a few months, is enough to clear up thrush completely. Even when you start taking it again, it may not return. It may go forever.

IUDs

The Pill is not the only method of contraception that can have a disastrous effect on a woman's health. Intra-uterine devices (IUDs for short) are second only to the Pill in preventing pregnancy effectively. They have not been in wide use for long enough for us to know exactly how harmful they may be. If the IUD has been incorrectly inserted, the uterus may be perforated. It then becomes possible for the IUD to slip out of the womb, through a perforation in the abdominal cavity, where it can cause pelvic inflammatory disease (PID). If pregnancy occurs while the IUD is in place, it may cause a miscarriage, accompanied by infection. There is also an increased risk that a fertilized ovum will become implanted in the Fallopian tube.

Less extreme side-effects of the IUD include heavy periods and bleeding between periods. Allergic skin reactions may occur in IUD users.

Because of the increased risk of vaginal or uterine infections that is associated with the use of IUDs, women who are prone to thrush should avoid them at all costs. The heavy bleeding that may be caused by this method of contraception, and the bleeding between periods provoke thrush.

If you suffer from thrush and feel that it may be related to your IUD, talk about it with your doctor and try to change to another form of contraceptive as soon as possible. On the other hand, if you use the Pill as a method of contraception and your doctor has recommended that you change to an IUD because of thrush, be very wary. Both the Pill and an IUD can be responsible for bringing about fungal infections and neither should really be looked on as an alternative to the other.

Antibiotics

Many women, and men too, experience an attack of thrush when they are taking, or have just finished, a course of antibiotic tablets. This is because antibiotics cause certain changes inside the body that make it easier for yeast organisms to take hold.

The term 'antibiotic' means life-destroying. It is applied to drugs containing chemicals that are obtained from micro-organisms (moulds, for example). They work by stopping the growth of 'bad' germs and eventually killing them, but they can have adverse effects, too.

Most broad-spectrum antibiotics kill a huge number of bacteria in the body, including those that are not particularly harmful. In other words, they kill the good germs along with the bad, but they do not affect yeasts. Without enough of the 'good' bacteria left in the immune system to keep them in check, the yeasts multiply out of all proportion. This is called an overgrowth, or *superinfection*. An overgrowth of yeast or *Candida* is often found in the intestines after a course of antibiotics, so the best way to avoid this is to avoid antibiotics completely.

If you get thrush when you take antibiotics, always ask your doctor, or whoever has prescribed them, if there is an alternative treatment. For some illnesses, there may well be. If your antibiotics are absolutely necessary, prepare for thrush before it begins. Ask for a prescription for an oral thrush medication (see Chapter 5) to take just after you have finished your course of antibiotics and/or use pessaries at the same time. If you use pessaries alone, however, it is more than likely that the thrush will recur.

By taking thrush medication while you are on antibiotics, you automatically lessen the chances of an attack getting a hold within the body. In people who are not particularly prone to thrush, such precautions will probably be enough to prevent it developing, but for anyone who has, or has had a *Candida* problem, antibiotics spell trouble. This is particularly true for anyone caught in the vicious cycle of cystitis and thrush.

Cystitis

Cystitis is yet another blight on womankind and female sexuality. Together with thrush, it is one of, if not *the*, most common infection to burden women, which is why a book such as this cannot deal with both in full. However, some information about cystitis must be included here. Cystitis and thrush are very much related with one another as urinary infections may often stem from fungal ones, and a lot of women who experience cystitis suffer from frequent thrush attacks, too, and vice versa. In general, the methods of preventing cystitis are the same as those that tend to keep thrush at bay. These are mentioned later on in this book in Chapter 11. If you suffer from both cystitis and thrush, then it is important to read these parts of the book.

True cystitis occurs when the urethra or bladder becomes infected. Today, many doctors use the term to cover an inflammation of the bladder and all sorts of urinary problems. This ambiguity concerning cystitis is not altogether surprising. When you have a bladder infection, you feel as though you want to go to the lavatory every few minutes, alhough there may be little or no urine to pass. When you do urinate, the urine burns and stings unbearably and there may be blood present (haematuria). Some women whose bladders are *inflamed* rather than infected — perhaps from vigorous sexual intercourse — experience similar symptoms to these, with the exception of haematuria. With each visit to the lavatory, the strain of forcing oneself to urinate has a harmful effect on the urethra. Minute tears occur in its lining so that each trickle of urine along the urethra is agonizing. Whether or not an infection was present originally seems, at this stage, to be of little importance. In any case, with the urethra in a state such as this, an infection is very likely to arise unless the sufferer seeks help.

Escherichia coliform (E. coli) is the germ that causes most bladder infections. It is a natural inhabitant of the bowel, and it causes no problems there. It is only when it finds its way into the urethra that trouble begins. It does not take long for the infection to reach the bladder. From there it may then travel up the ureters — the tubes that carry urine from the kidneys to the bladder. If the infection is allowed to progress this far, the kidneys will be affected. A kidney infection is serious, even dangerous. This is why it is important not to ignore the early symptoms of cystitis in the hope that they will vanish of their own accord.

Doctors treat most cases of cystitis with antibiotic drugs. These are very efficient and symptoms usually disappear after a few days. It is important to continue the full course of treatment — just as it is when you are treated for thrush.

Although cystitis may or may not be related to an infection, often it will only clear up with antibiotics. Sometimes, if the trouble is caught in its earliest stages, it is possible to cure it yourself. This involves drinking enormous amounts of liquid, preferably water, usually about 300 ml (½ pint) every 20 minutes. However, the intense pain that is associated with cystitis — and all its miseries — is often too much to bear. Antibiotics are then taken when they are not strictly necessary, and the symptoms go away. Antibiotics may *appear* to be a lifesaver, but, unfortunately, this is not so, as many women have found out. The treatment taken to cure cystitis often results in bringing on an attack of thrush, especially in those who are prone to fungal infections. The fungus, having taken a hold in the vagina, then finds its way into the urethra, and irritates the tissues there that are in the process of healing. The scars in the lining of the urethra open up so that it feels as though the cystitis has returned. Thrush, therefore, can actually bring on another attack of cystitis. In treating the cystitis, the thrush will probably return, and so on.

The vicious circle of cystitis and thrush can be very nasty and very difficult to break. Even if you suffer from cystitis and, as yet, have not been afflicted with the added distress of thrush, the possibilities of this merry-go-round are ever present.

> In a way, thrush for me is sex linked. I am prone to urinary tract infections, which I invariably get if I don't pass water immediately after sex. The doctor then treats me with antibiotics, which in turn cause thrush; so the two go hand in hand for me.

> I find cystitis and thrush often occur one after the other, the antibiotics for the cystitis causing the thrush to thrive. Most courses of antibiotics have this effect (especially the 'tetracyclines'). Also, if I'm run down, the thrush tends to return.

> I have suffered from recurrent thrush for several years. Unfortunately, I have also suffered from a urological complaint requiring surgery three years ago, which has left me with a tendency to cystitis, in particular following intercourse. This requires regular treatment with antibiotics, which in turn leads to another attack of thrush.

If you are suffering from what seems like cystitis, always visit your doctor. Insist that your urine is tested to see whether an infection is present and wait for the results before taking antibiotics — remember, they may not be necessary. In the meantime, try to achieve an effective cure for yourself by drinking plenty of water and urinating frequently so that your system is constantly being flushed through. Mixing a little bicarbonate of soda (an alkalizing agent) into your drinks helps to ease the burning. Stay indoors and try to keep as warm as possible. Placing a hot water bottle against your stomach will help to relieve the pain. This treatment will be more effective if it is begun as the first sensations of an attack are felt.

There are several over-the-counter remedies now available for cystitis. They should be viewed as pain relievers rather than permanent cures. They cannot cure a bacterial infection of cystitis, but they may help stop the burning sensations until you can get to a doctor. Your chemist should be able to advise you which of them will be the most suitable for you.

If you think you can cure your attack of cystitis without a doctor's medicine — this may be relevant for women who suffer from cystitis again and again, who can well recognize the symptoms — try to do so. Alternative treatments to antibiotics include drinking Mis. Pot. Cit, diluted with plenty of water. Mis. Pot. Cit is an old-fashioned remedy for urinary infections. It contains a compound of potassium citrate, and works well, despite its vile taste, because it helps to stop the urine from burning. Mis. Pot. Cit is available over the counter at any good chemist's. Similarly, tablets to relieve cystitis can be bought from healthfood shops.

If you are in any doubt about why you have cystitis or are at all worried, it is always best to ask your doctor's advice. If your doctor feels it is imperative that your cystitis should be treated with antibiotics, and you are prone to thrush, ask for a course of thrush treatment that you can use at the same time as a preventative measure.

On a final note, remember that where both cystitis and thrush are concerned, self-help will always be the best remedy, and by following the advice set out in this book their tendency to recur can be considerably lessened.

The menopause

Strictly speaking the term 'menopause' means the final period. It is the time when menstruation permanently ceases. For many women, however, this process takes place gradually and is accompanied by a lot of unpleasant symptoms or side-effects.

As a woman reaches the menopause, her ovaries stop producing a monthly ovum (egg) and cease to produce the female sex hormones, oestrogen and progesterone. The gradual decrease in the supply of these hormones causes changes to occur in the body. The vagina becomes narrower, shorter and hard. The loss of moisture and elasticity in the vagina is called *vaginal atrophy*, and it happens because of the greatly reduced secretions of the vaginal walls. This, in turn, can lead to an increased susceptibility to vaginal infection. When the soft inner surfaces of the vagina are damaged — for example, after intercourse without sufficient lubrication — it becomes even more vulnerable. Tears and abrasions provide a place for otherwise harmless organisms to grow out of all proportion.

Hormone replacement therapy (HRT) with oestrogen can relieve vaginal dryness, possibly preventing vaginitis and other infections, like thrush. Oestrogen creams such as Dienoestrol, applied directly to the vagina, may also be beneficial.

Hormonal imbalance

When the balance of the hormones oestrogen and progesterone changes, as it does during the menopause, the secretions of the walls of the vagina and cervix are affected. In fact, in women who have periods, the level of these hormones is continually changing, so that the amount and consistency of a vaginal discharge varies throughout the menstrual cycle. The discharge may increase at ovulation or before a period. The bacteria within the vagina are well adjusted to these patterns and usually no problems occur. The *lactobacilli* convert glycogen in the vaginal fluid into lactic acid. They maintain the vagina's acidity at just the right level and thus prevent the growth of harmful organisms.

However, if the level of either one or both of these hormones, oestrogen and progesterone, changes dramatically, the delicate pH balance of the vagina will be affected. The *lactobacilli* are unable to function properly and infections can easily flare up. A hormonal imbalance may be contributing to a recurrent thrush problem. Only a thorough medical investigation will either confirm or eliminate this as a possible cause. If you suspect that this is the reason you are suffering, ask your doctor's advice.

Men

You can catch thrush from someone else. About four out of ten cases of thrush are passed on to a sexual partner. This is why it is important to practise 'safe sex' and use a condom when you have thrush. Most people find that it is best to avoid sex altogether until the thrush has cleared up to prevent infecting your partner and possibly reinfecting yourself!

Some men seem to have more akaline semen than others, and this can be enough to trigger off an attack of thrush. Apart from changing your lover, there are other less drastic ways to resolve this problem! A cream like Aci-jel (see Chapter 5) can be used as a lubricant during sexual intercourse. This may counteract the alkaline effect of the semen. Barrier methods of contraception, such as a condom or cap, are obviously a help, especially if used in conjunction with spermicidal jellies and foams. These tend to wash out germs and may stop them from growing (see Chapter 6). The Pill and an IUD give no protection against infection and may possibly encourage fungal growth (see pages 13–15).

> I was a thrush sufferer for 12 years. My ex-husband also suffered. I now believe that I was not chemically compatible with my husband. During the years that I had it, I would have thrush for two weeks of every four. After the birth of my first child, I was completely free of thrush, but, on resuming intercourse at three months, I got it immediately again. I used every pessary on the market, visited doctors, VD clinics, etc. I thought I had it for life, thankfully not. It makes you wonder if I'd stayed with my ex-husband if I'd have ended up with cancer.

> I've suffered since 1979, and experienced about six attacks a year. Now I get thrush every two weeks. I must admit it seems sexually transmitted in my case because, if I abstain, I don't get thrush. I did suggest to my doctor that perhaps I was allergic to my husband, but this was poo-poohed! But I got married in 1979, which was when it all started.

Diet

Diabetic women are highly susceptible to thrush. This is because the sugar content in their blood stream is too high. The amount of glycogen secreted by the walls of the vagina increases to such an extent that the bacteria there, whose job it is to convert glycogen into lactic acid, simply cannot cope. Sugar in the urine also gets deposited on the vulva, and so provides fungus with the sweet food it needs to thrive. Where there is sugar, thrush can grow and multiply.

Diet plays a vital role in the control of fungal infections for all of us, diabetic or not. It is important for two reasons:

- certain foods can actually *provoke* attacks — we need to know what these are, in which ways they are harmful and how we can avoid them
- by eating other foods, we can build up a *resistance* to fungal infections and actually protect our bodies.

Chapter 7 discusses diet in more detail; it is a complicated subject and needs to be carefully understood, so suffice it to say that it is important here.

Stress

Stress is not an illness. It is a symptom or, rather, a set of symptoms that occur when our bodies can no longer handle the rough treatment we have been giving them. Many minor complaints, like colds, migraines and backache are simply our body's reaction to stress. If we ignore these danger signals, more serious stress-related diseases develop. Thus, stress can be the cause of many illnesses – stomach ulcers, diabetes and heart disease, to name but a few.

The causes of stress may be psychological or physical, social or environmental. Marriage, divorce, sexual problems, the death of someone very close to us, and unemployment are psychological stress factors. Minor and/or serious injuries — even pregnancy — are conducive to stress. In fact, anything that puts undue pressure on us, presents us with emotional difficulties or anxiety, or upsets our everyday routine, can produce stress.

There are times when we all suffer from stress. However, the amount of stress the body can tolerate varies from person to person, so that we do not all react to stress in the same way. For reasons yet unknown, some human beings are better able to cope with pressure than others.

The worst thing about stress is that it can result in illness, which then subjects the body to more stress. Thrush is a stress-related disease. Recurrent thrush may be both stress-related and a cause of thrush in its own right. We worry when attacks stubbornly refuse to respond to treatment and we thus expose ourselves to more stress. This creates a vicious circle that can be extremely hard to break.

Avoiding stress is the simplest way to prevent thrush if you suspect that these are related. As there may be two or more factors contributing to a recurrent thrush problem, it is usually very difficult to identify stress as a bona fide cause. However, poor health, an inadequate diet, or generally being run down, may provoke an attack of thrush. By making sure that you have enough sleep, improve your diet, and learn to relax, you will increase your stress tolerance level and your resistance to any vaginal infection.

Why do people get oral thrush?

This chapter has dealt mainly with vaginal thrush. The vagina is similar to the mouth in many respects — it is dark, warm and wet — which is why thrush can crop up in either of these places. If you have thrush, you probably would not notice that you had also got it in your bowel and intestines, too.

Oral thrush is fairly unusual in healthy adults, but may be brought on by a course of antibiotics, sedatives or steroids. Inhaling corticosteroids can cause oral thrush, too.

Because their immune systems do not work properly, AIDS sufferers usually develop chronic thrush, often in their mouths (see Chapter 1). Ulcers and other lesions in the mouth can become infected with *Candida*. This is why people with false teeth sometimes develop oral thrush. Sore spots along the gums, irritated by dentures, can harbour pockets of *Candida*. If you suffer from oral thrush and you have false teeth, remember to sterilize your dentures regularly.

The vagina is protected by its mucus discharge and, in a similar way, the mouth is kept clean and healthy by the saliva. Saliva is an important weapon in protecting the mouth from disease. Using powerful mouthwashes can occasionally upset the mouth's eco system enough to cause an overgrowth of *Candida* there. If you want to gargle, use good old-fashioned salt in warm water!

3

Some other causes

Chapter 2 discussed some of the more obvious causes of thrush — antibiotics, the Pill, cervical eversion, pregnancy, illness, and hormonal changes and disorders. If you can attribute your attack of thrush to any of these causes then it is quite likely that the problem will completely disappear once the root cause has been removed.

If, however, the cause of your thrush infection is less apparent, it will be more difficult to effect a cure. It is often difficult to identify the cause of a recurrent thrush problem simply because there may be a combination of reasons for its existence. Recurrent thrush may be caused by an untreated infection elsewhere in the body, and/or be aggravated by one of many factors. Establishing just what these might be is usually a matter of trial and error. Sometimes this can only be done by eliminating certain things in your life — one by one — that may be possible causes of the problem. This chapter deals with the sorts of things that have become an accepted part of our everyday lives and yet can be so detrimental to our health.

Tights and tight trousers

All fungi thrive in warm and moist conditions. Fresh air circulating around the vulva (the outer genitals) is vital. It inhibits abnormal fungal growth. Years ago, when our grandmothers walked around in loose, cotton underclothes, thrush was a rarity. The advent of nylon and other man-made fabrics soon changed things. Synthetic fabrics retain moisture as the close-woven mesh of their fibres is too fine to allow normal circulating air to pass through it. By wearing nylon pants and tights, we are depriving the surface sex organs of the fresh air needed to keep them dry, and to keep thrush and other vaginal infections at bay.

Nylon underwear and tights do not absorb moisture, so that when the mixture of sweat and the vagina's own natural secretions begins to accumulate, the crotch becomes a very hot and sticky place. In fact, it becomes an ideal breeding ground for thrush and other harmful bacteria.

Tight trousers can also provoke an attack of thrush because they provide a barrier to the air circulation around the genital area, and trap the sweat from the crotch. Tight jeans also rub together when you walk. The heat generated from this friction can only make the situation worse. Layers of heavy denim are bad enough on their own. When they are worn over nylon tights and pants, the effect is potentially disastrous.

Thrush may be caused by tight trousers and/or underwear made from synthetic fabrics. Both make an existing thrush problem much worse and may be the reason why attacks are so difficult to clear up. One of the first rules of self-help for thrush is not to wear nylon plants or tights. Always wear cotton pants – or, better still, none at all, when this is possible. Throw your tight trousers away. Wear loose-fitting trousers or, if you cannot do without jeans, wear skirts on alternate days, and never, never wear nylon pants and nylon tights under tight trousers. This lethal combination is an open invitation to thrush. A thrush attack can build up in a matter of minutes under such conditions.

It is an especially good idea to avoid trousers when you are recovering from an attack, say in the two to three weeks after finishing a course of pessaries. Wearing no pants at all will obviously help here, too. A longish skirt will hide all! If you do not feel comfortable like this, you could at least forgo your undies in the privacy of your own house.

Soaps and washing powders

Cotton underwear should always be boiled — in plain water. Thrush spores are only killed by boiling, and washing powders also contain harsh chemicals. These can irritate tender areas like the vagina. They can also kill off the valuable natural ecological balance in the genital area and, therefore, make it easier for the 'bad' bacteria to take hold. Medicated soaps have a similar effect. They act as an irritant. They are most unnecessary around the vagina as it secretes its own fluids as cleansing agents, keeping it beautifully clean. Washing should help nature, not destroy it. For this reason it is best to cleanse the vagina by pouring cold, pure water over the perineum, but even then it is not advisable to do this more than once a day. If you suspect that your thrush infection is related to *Candida* from the bowel, always wash after passing a stool. Use a little pure soap around the anus and rinse it off with ordinary water. The only other time you actually need to wash the genital area is after intercourse. Pouring cold water over the vulva helps to prevent urinary infections by washing away germs before they can reach the urethral opening.

Baths

While bathing in salt water can be beneficial in treating some vaginal infections, soaking for any length of time in a hot bath can be enough to trigger off an attack of thrush. This is why showers are better for women prone to the infection. Salt baths are recommended for the treatment of non-specific vaginitis when there is very little else that can be done. If you suffer from recurrent thrush, avoid baths. If you must bathe, make it quick and preferably in only a few inches of cool or lukewarm water. Never have a bath during a full-scale attack of thrush.

Vaginal deodorants

Vaginal deodorants are an unnecessary hazard, irritating the mucous membranes and possibly provoking an attack of thrush. In any case they cannot work properly as they do not affect germs inside the vagina. Instead, they make it dry and itchy and can cause allergic reactions. Bubble baths and antiseptics should not be used for the same reasons. Perfumed soaps are to be avoided, too, as they kill off the natural bacteria in the vagina in much the same way as antibiotics do.

Sanitary protection

There are now so many different kinds of sanitary protection products on the market that it is difficult to know where to begin when you want to buy some. However, your choice of sanitary protection is all-important if you suffer from thrush — your choice might actually be the cause.

Tampons

Whether or not tampons are a cause of thrush is not fully known. What is clear, however, is that most women are particularly prone to thrush just before, during or just after a period. Because blood is alkaline, it makes the vagina susceptible to *Candida*. If a tampon is left for too long in the vagina, the wad of fibre can become a breeding ground for vaginal infections. Few women could deny that it is easier to forget they have a tampon inside their vaginas than it is to forget that they are using a sanitary towel.

The sorts of fibres most tampons contain are also slightly suspect, particularly those that claim a super absorbency. Most tampons are made from varying combinations of cotton and rayon, depending on the price of raw materials. Some contain a percentage of carboxymethyl cellulose fibres for extra absorbency. Super absorbency tampons are rarely necessary except at night, when you keep a tampon in place for a much longer period of time. They tend to have an unnatural drying effect on the vagina, making it more susceptible to thrush and other infections.

Towels may or may not be an alternative sanitary protection for thrush sufferers. If you have recurrent thrush and you use tampons, try sanitary towels to see if the problem improves. Wearing a sanitary towel at night is at least preferable to using a super absorbency tampon.

Sanitary towels

The first commercial disposable sanitary towel was made in the 1880s. It is reported to have cost the same price as a pair of shoes so, not surprisingly, very few women could actually afford to buy them. In fact, until the mid 1950s, most women in Britain still wore their own reusable sanitary towels. They made and washed these themselves, just as their mothers and grandmothers had done before them, and just as millions of women in other parts of the world still do today.

In recent years, the sanitary towel — a thick pad of cotton or synthetic fibres — has become progressively slimmer and 'super absorbent'. These towels contain chemicals such as *polyacrylate gels*, also found in disposable nappies, that can absorb many times their own weight in liquid. The gels do not allow the liquid to flow out again, even under pressure.

Super slim (absorbent) towels are claimed to be perfectly safe, but workers manufacturing the gels risk health problems. If the gels come into contact with the eyes, they can cause irritation or even temporary damage. If they are inhaled, they may cause lung problems.

Unfortunately no independent research exists right now as to the effects of the new super absorbent towels on women's health. It is quite likely that these — and all other sanitary towels that come backed with leak-proof plastic — prevent air from circulating around the vulva and so are best avoided by thrush sufferers.

Pant liners

Women do not need pant liners — after all, we wear underwear to keep our bodies' secretions away from our clothes! Unfortunately, pant liners have been marketed as hygienic essentials so that many women feel that they *should* need them. We are told that a vaginal discharge is unpleasant and a problem. It is not — it is normal and actually keeps the vagina clean and healthy. On the other hand, a smelly or offensive vaginal discharge *is* a sign of a problem — an infection. However, in this case, wearing pant liners will not make an infection any better and, indeed, could make the problem worse. An advertisement for pant liners that unfortunately would never get past the client might run like this: if you need a pant liner, you should see your doctor!

Fresh air is essential for keeping the vagina healthy; by wearing pads day in, day out you will be preventing air from circulating around the vulva, making it a hot-house for infection. Many women suffer from mild stress incontinence, for example when coughing, and so they use pant liners every day. Again this is unnecessary. Mild stress incontinence is easily curable by a visit to the doctor.

Chemically impregnated towels, tampons and pant liners can irritate the delicate mucous membranes of the vagina. One of the most important rules of women's health really ought to be 'Never put anything inside your vagina that you wouldn't put into your mouth'. Never, ever use tampons or sanitary towels that contain deodorants. Avoid tampons that have plastic applicators as these have sharp, pointed teeth, which can nick or cut the delicate skin in or around the vagina, and so cause an infection to occur. Be particularly careful if you have an IUD fitted as fibres from a tampon may catch on the string of the IUD and this may give rise to infections.

In the UK, the Women's Environmental Network has campaigned successfully for chlorine-free sanitary protection products and health warnings on packets of tampons. For accurate, clear, up-to-date information about the chemicals in sanitary towels and tampons contact them at the address given on page 115.

Alternatives to tampons and towels

Natural sponges are an alternative to conventional sanitary protection. Although they are not as convenient to use as towels or tampons, they are certainly a lot cheaper. Sponges can be bought quite cheaply from most chemists.

It is best to choose one that has tiny holes. Attach a longish thread of cotton to the sponge to make removal easier. Some women find that they do not need a string, but others do, although the sponge could never be inserted so high that your fingers could not reach it. Soak the sponge in water and squeeze it so that it is slightly damp. Once the sponge is in place, it should be treated like a normal tampon as it has the same absorbency. When you change the sponge (every two or three hours), do not throw it away. Simply wash it in cool, running water, squeeze and then insert into the vagina again. Although there are no problems of disposal you will need to find a lavatory with a washbasin at hand. Buy two sponges so that you always have a spare in case of emergencies.

Sponges are also useful for applying acidic solutions to the vagina. They can be soaked in diluted vinegar or lemon juice, yogurt, and herbal preparations and then put into place to ward off thrush attacks (see Chapter 6, Self-help remedies).

A word of warning

Toxic shock syndrome (TSS) is a rare, but, none the less, very real threat to women. TSS is defined as a severe infection of the blood. The blood becomes poisoned by toxins produced by strains of the *Staphyloccus aureus* bacteria.

This bacteria is normally harmless and is often found in and around the vagina. Certain conditions trigger this bacteria to produce the deadly toxins of TSS, but no one knows for sure exactly what these conditions are. Almost half of all the cases identified have been menstruating young women wearing tampons. It is thought that tampons provide a breeding ground for the bacteria, menstrual blood providing the nutrients the bacteria need to grow. Super absorbent tampons have also been blamed; they can dry and damage the vaginal walls and so make it easier for the toxins to pass through the mucous membranes into the bloodstream.

TSS produces symptoms such as:

- sudden high temperature
- vomiting
- headache

- confusion
- sunburn-like rash

Younger women seem to be most at risk. Probably because their immune systems are less developed, their bodies are rapidly overwhelmed by the toxins. However, any woman who has these symptoms during her period should get medical help immediately!

All types and brands of tampons have been linked with TSS especially the higher absorbency ones. To minimize the risk, change your tampon every two to four hours and do not wear tampons overnight. Natural sponges may also carry the risks of TSS as they are worn internally.

The Green movement and general concern for the environment has made the idea of reusable sanitary towels attractive to many women. In the USA, there are several brands of washable sanitary towels on the market. In the UK, Ecofem washable sanitary towels are available from Ganmill Limited (for their address, see page 115).

4

Getting medical help

If you suspect you have thrush and you have never had it before, then you should visit a doctor. It is vital to get a proper diagnosis and medical help as soon as you can. After all, you may not have thrush at all — there are other genital infections that share the same symptoms (see Chapter 8) — and the longer an infection has to develop, the more serious it becomes. If you allow thrush to persist untreated, it will simply become more irritating and painful. The maddening itch associated with thrush can be embarrassing as well as infuriating — there is nothing worse than needing to scratch yourself when in public!

Modern society has left us ashamed of our bodies — not to mention our bodily functions, and there is still a great deal of social stigma attached to venereal disease and to our sex organs in general. When we think we have a genital infection we may be, wrongly, afraid to go to a doctor.

GPs and thrush

Until recently, most women who suffered from thrush *had* to go to a doctor for help. Fortunately, this is no longer the case. Antifungal pessaries and vaginal creams are now available over the counter, which means they can be bought at your local chemist. This has helped many recurrent thrush sufferers. These patients recognize the symptoms of thrush from previous attacks and can quickly seek out treatment for themselves.

Recurrent sufferers will be familiar with using the pessaries available at chemists. They will sigh with relief at the mere thought that getting the medication which can rid them of their painful thrush problem does not require getting past their doctor's receptionist! But, and this is a very big BUT, you should definitely visit your GP before buying a course of treatment if:

- you are, or think you might be, pregnant
- you notice any abnormal or irregular vaginal bleeding or a bloodstained discharge

- you might have caught another sexually transmitted disease, from a new or regular partner
- you have vaginal sores, ulcers or blisters
- you have any pain in your abdomen or difficulty passing urine.

Obviously you should also visit a doctor if you have used a thrush preparation to no effect or if this treatment seems to have made your symptoms worse.

This chapter is all about doctors. It details where you should go for either an initial diagnosis or an expert's opinion. It will tell you what to expect, wherever you choose to go for help, and, hopefully, will set you on your way to saying goodbye to thrush — forever!

Everyone living in the UK, on a permanent or temporary basis, is entitled to register themselves with a general practitioner (GP). You do not need to pay for an appointment. This service is financed by the National Insurance contributions that we make throughout our lives, in sickness and in health. In other countries, where a National Health Service does not exist, visiting a doctor is not so easy. Nor are the appointments 'free'. When many visits have to be made frequently — as in the case of the sufferer of recurrent thrush — this can be quite costly. However, the price of ill health pales in comparison with the emotional and psychological trial of repeated visits to a doctor. Arranging one's life around surgery appointments is hardly fun, especially if each visit has little or no result.

You can help to make your visits more pleasant and more fruitful. If you are suffering from an attack of thrush, try to see a doctor at the earliest opportunity. As it is virtually impossible to predict when an attack will flare up, surgeries operating on a non-appointment basis are better for women prone to thrush. If you *have* to wait several days before a doctor can see you, though, you can ease your discomfort by keeping the vulva as clean and dry as possible. Wear loose, cotton clothing and avoid jeans, tights and baths. The itching and soreness may be relieved by applying witch hazel to the vulva with swabs of cotton wool. A mild lanolin cream will help to relieve the symptoms until they can be properly treated. Always be wary of proprietary brand creams that claim to stop embarrassing itches. Itching is a symptom of thrush, so do not ignore it!

Many women try to cure thrush with pessaries that they may have left over from previous attacks. Do not be tempted to do this unless you are sure that you have enough to completely clear the infection. Half a course of treatment is worse, in the long run, than no treatment at all. A few pessaries temporarily mask the symptoms and may result in negative swab tests.

Before you arrive at the doctor's, be prepared for an internal examination. This is the only way the doctor will be able to make an accurate diagnosis. If your doctor does not want to examine you, ask them to do so anyway. It is possible for other conditions to be present in the vagina as well as thrush. The symptoms of thrush can be mistaken for other diseases, and vice versa. Insist on a proper examination before you accept any treatment.

If you are found to have a genital infection, your doctor should prescribe some form of treatment, or may refer you to a special clinic or to a gynaecologist. Always ask the doctor what they are giving you, how to take it and if it is likely to have any side-effects. If you are unhappy about your treatment, say so!

Before your visit, make a note of any questions you have about thrush. It is unlikely that you will remember all of the things you want to ask once you are sitting in the surgery. Tell the doctor if you do not understand anything they say and mention anything you feel might help the doctor. The more they know about your thrush problem, the more chance you will both have of overcoming it.

If you suffer from recurrent thrush, it would be wise to ask your doctor if they will give you a repeat prescription for pessaries and cream. This will save you and your doctor a lot of time in appointment visits. It also means that, as soon as you spot an infection, you can start to treat it straight away. You should also use the pessaries at high-risk times – inserting one pessary into the vagina each night during the last few days of your period, for example. If you are particularly susceptible to thrush, get your doctor to write 'Not to be given antibiotics, unless essential' on your medical file. This will ensure that you are not advised to take these drugs (when they are not strictly necessary, in the case of a sore throat, for example) on those occasions when you are not seen by your regular doctor.

Always try to make something positive happen from a visit: if pessaries are not working for you, do not allow yourself to be sent away with yet another course. If you are having little success with your doctor, ask them to refer you to a specialist. A persistent thrush problem should be thoroughly investigated. Should your doctor admit that they cannot do anything more for you, get them to refer you to someone who can.

> . . . The important thing is that now I know how to cope with subsequent thrush attacks, which, unfortunately, I admit are likely to occur. I have confidence in my doctor and her wish to help rather than simply sign a prescription for more pessaries. My advice to other sufferers, especially those people experiencing a first attack, is to go to their doctor promptly . . . As a pharmacy student I would advise others that their local pharmacist will be able to suggest a suitable cream, not to cure thrush but to relieve itching and soothe inflammation before an appointment at the doctor's can be made.

Women doctors may be more helpful as they may have had the same infection themselves. If you are unhappy with the treatment you have been receiving, it may be worth changing your doctor.

Special clinics

If you think that you have thrush, you can go to a special clinic. These offer one of the best facilities for the accurate diagnosis and prompt treatment of all genital infections. Most general hospitals have special clinics attached to them and they are sometimes known by other names. These include Department of Genito-urinary Medicine or Department of Venereology and Sexually Transmitted Disease, or STD clinics.

In 1991, a total of 634 438 new patients were seen in special clinics in the UK. Of these, nearly 60 000 were treated for thrush. Although these clinics still have some social stigmas attached to them, only 58 per cent of patients actually had a sexually transmitted infection.

In the UK, anyone can attend a special clinic without being referred by their own doctor — a situation that does not exist in some other countries. (In the USA, Australia and New Zealand, for example, women with thrush would not normally be accepted for treatment.) Most special clinics now operate on an appointment basis so that it is best to telephone before you arrive. The address of your nearest clinic can be obtained from a family planning clinic, or by telephoning, or asking at your local hospital.

Many people feel nervous about attending a special clinic, but the experience should not be a traumatic one. The atmosphere is relaxed and friendly. The staff try hard to put their patients at ease. Complete confidentiality is assured. Remember that the doctors here are experts and they will be able to answer any of the questions you might wish to ask them. You, yourself, must also be prepared to answer all of the doctor's questions with absolute honesty. Your answers will help the clinic to make a correct diagnosis. You will be asked for some basic information about yourself: name, address, age and so on. The clinic will also want to know about any recent sexual contacts, any contraception you are using and a little about your past medical history.

You will then be examined by a doctor. You will be asked to undress from the waist downwards and lie on a couch, with your legs apart. The doctor will insert a speculum into your vagina. This holds the walls of the vagina open so that they can get a clear view of the walls and the cervix. Swabs from the vagina and cervix will be taken. Anal and urethral swabs may also be taken. Cervical smears are usually performed as a matter of routine. You will also be given a blood test.

It is possible that you will be asked for a urine sample. For this reason, it is sensible to have a full bladder when you attend. Some clinics will ask new patients not to pass water for at least two hours before their appointment.

The vaginal and cervical swabs are examined on a slide and analysed under a microscope so that a diagnosis can be made on the spot. If you have thrush, the doctor should be able to tell you so immediately and treatment can begin at once. Sometimes, the fungi are not instantly detectable. Swabs will be sent to the laboratory and you may have to wait up to a week for the results to come through.

The policy of most genito-urinary clinics is only to treat what they find. In effect, this means that even if you have all the symptoms of thrush, they will not prescribe anything until they have their own microscopic evidence. This attitude may be frustrating for women convinced that they have thrush. It does have its advantages, however. For example, a doctor will often take the patient at their word and will treat that patient for the condition that they complain of without carrying out a proper examination. Drugs are powerful chemicals, which is why they are so effective, but, where there is no infection, they can be positively harmful, possibly provoking thrush.

> On many occasions, believing that my thrush had returned, I would go to a special clinic where their routine tests would have confirmed *Candida* if it were present. Because they did not, I had

> to leave things to calm down a bit on their own. And each time, the non-specific infection — which indeed had all the symptoms of thrush — disappeared after a few days. Had I used the strong medication contained in pessaries I would have further disturbed the flora in the vagina, perhaps even bringing on an attack of thrush. In fact, I am sure that the latter happened because of this on many occasions.

Whether or not you are found to be suffering from a genital infection, you will be asked to return for routine follow-up tests. It is essential to attend. It is also important to ask your sexual partner or partners to attend. An asymptomatic male partner may be carrying an infection. Men can harbour thrush spores under the foreskin. Reinfection will occur as soon as sexual contact begins again.

There is a strong link between recurrent NSU and thrush. This is a much more serious disease as, left untreated, it can have severe consequences (see page 4). For this reason alone, sexually active women with thrush should ensure that any male contact is also treated.

The gynaecologist

Recurrent thrush problems should always be fully investigated, preferably by a gynaecologist. Women in the UK must be referred by their doctor. There may be a waiting list for an appointment. If you have to wait several months, ask your doctor to continue treating you for thrush until you see the specialist.

Gynaecologists are trained to deal with disorders of women's sexual and reproductive organs. You will be examined internally. You may be asked for a urine sample and given a smear test. As with an ordinary doctor's appointment, it is wise to write down a list of things you wish to discuss with your gynaecologist. Although they can only treat their patients with the same drugs that doctors prescribe, they will investigate a persistent gynaecological problem. They may identify its cause or any underlying factors, previously overlooked by your doctor. For example, an irritation of the cervix can be a source of recurrent thrush. A gynaecologist will be able to treat this and, in doing so, may rid you of thrush.

Well Woman clinics

A Well Woman clinic is a clinic where any woman can go to have a check-up on, and a chat about, her health. They were set up to help women with problems and medical conditions that are often neglected by other parts of the Health Service: cystitis, depression, tiredness, problems connected with periods and the menopause and many others, including, of course, thrush. They offer a unique service in health care because the staff (all women) have plenty of time to listen to their patients — with sympathy and understanding. They try to provide information, advice and help so that women can learn more about their bodies and their health. Unlike other clinics that only see patients when they are sick, Well Woman centres will help women who are in good health and who want to stay that way. Great emphasis is put on the prevention and early detection of disease.

Well Woman clinics believe that your emotional health is just as important as a physical problem. They will examine you and give you advice and information about any symptoms that are worrying you. Some of the simple tests that can be done here include those to check your blood pressure, urine, weight, height, and eyesight. You may also be given a cervical smear test, breast and/or vaginal examination. The clinics also provide a counselling service if you have personal problems or family worries that you need to talk about. Well Woman clinics are good news because they offer more positive support towards mental and social good health.

When you arrive at a Well Woman clinic, you will be asked to fill in a questionnaire about yourself and your general health and well-being. This gives the clinic an overall picture of your health and helps them to isolate the areas that are worrying you. You may also be given another questionnaire to fill in and return to the clinic after your visit, to tell them whether the clinic has been helpful and how they can improve it.

You will then see a worker. She will help you to complete the questionnaire. She will have a long talk with you to find out what problems you have and how the clinic might be able to help. She will give you any advice she has and may do some tests. She may want you to see another worker who has a more specialized knowledge — a social worker, marriage guidance consellor or another type of counsellor — or she may refer you immediately to the clinic doctor.

Well Woman clinics are excellent places to go if you suffer from recurrent thrush. Although the staff cannot give you a prescription, they will examine you to see whether you actually have an infection and refer you to a doctor for treatment. The clinics will advise you on treatments available through your doctor and explain what these entail. Well Woman clinics will also give you the emotional support that all thrush sufferers so desperately need.

At the end of your visit, the clinic will give you a card. This will be your record of the tests you have had there. If they suggest some simple treatment for you to follow or if the doctor is counselling you for a personal problem, they may suggest you come back to the clinic again to see if your problems are getting better.

At present, Well Woman clinics in the UK are few and far between. If you want to find out whether there is one in your area, ask at your hospital. Alternatively, your District Health Authority or Community Health Council will be able to tell you where the nearest clinic is.

Women's health centres

In countries such as Australia and New Zealand, women's health centres operate on a similar basis to Well Woman clinics. Many of these have now formed self-help groups to combat vaginal infections like thrush and are helping to remove the ignorance associated with genital diseases in general.

Herbalist medicine

If conventional treatments fail, treatment by a qualified herbal practitioner is always worth considering. Rather than relieving the symptoms of disease with drugs, vaccines or synthetic substances, herbal medicine uses remedies from natural sources to restore good health.

During the initial consultation, all aspects of the patient's health are examined. Treatment for recurrent thrush will invariably include a change of diet as well as the use of external poultices with potent antifungal agents. Internal medicines to improve pelvic circulation and restore normal tone to the reproductive organs will also be given.

The National Institute of Medical Herbalists is the oldest professional organization of Herbal Practitioners. A full list of its registered members can be obtained from the address given on page 114.

Homeopathy

Homeopathy is a combination of natural healing and medical science. Homeopathic cures encourage the body to fight disease. Treatments are given that would produce the same symptoms in a healthy person as those the patient complains of. By putting more of the disease into the body, the body's natural defences are further stimulated to resist the infection. Obviously, at first, the symptoms of the illness will worsen, but homeopathy works on the theory that what causes something can also cure it.

Before a diagnosis is made, the homeopathic doctor will examine the patient in depth. Great emphasis is placed on life-style, diet and the condition of the patient's health generally. Their personality and emotions will also be considered.

Borax tablets are often recommended as a treatment for thrush. These tablets may be hard or soft and taste sweet. It is important to remember not to touch the tablets with your hands as this is believed to render them ineffective. Tip the tablets into the cap of the container then drop them into your mouth. Allow about 30 minutes without food or drink before and after taking homeopathic medicines. Coffee, peppermint and eucalyptus oil (Olbas oil) are antidotes to homeopathic medicines, so avoid them when being treated in this way.

> About three years ago, I had thrush on and off for nearly 12 months. Nothing my doctor gave me worked so I decided to visit a homeopath.
>
> The homeopath gave me some Hydrastis Calendula pessaries. They were bright yellow and very gooey, but they really worked!
>
> I've had a few attacks since then and I've always used the same treatment. They clear up my thrush a treat. Now I tend to consult my homeopath about all my health problems.

Homeopathic medicine is now available, in the UK, on the National Health Service. There are five homeopathic hospitals — in London, Glasgow, Liverpool, Bristol and Tunbridge Wells — as well as numerous homeopathic clinics. If you think homeopathy may be able to help you, contact the British Homeopathic Association at the address for them given on page 114, enclosing a stamped addressed envelope, for a list of homeopathic doctors.

In the UK, homeopathic medicines are available over the counter at specialist chemists or by post from several manufacturers (the companies given on page 114 make a full range of homeopathic medicines and despatch them by mail order).

5
Treating thrush

This chapter outlines the various types of medication used to treat thrush. There are lots of different brands available and if you have had thrush several times, you may well be familiar with them all. Some of the creams and pessaries most effective in treating thrush can be bought over the counter at a pharmacy. But almost all of the medications necessary to treat recurrent thrush are available on prescription only.

All of the treatments outlined in this chapter usually work quickly and effectively. A short course can relieve an attack of thrush within days. Each doctor/clinic will have their own favourite. Similarly, after repeated infections, the thrush sufferer will begin to know which brand works best for them. If you are prescribed a medicine that you have tried before and have had little success with, do not be afraid to ask for an alternative.

Pessaries and creams

The most effective way to treat thrush is with creams (applied to the infected areas) and pessaries. In many cases, these work well. Cream helps to check the fungal growth and, eventually, kill it. Women should use it around the perineum and external labia. Men should apply the cream under the foreskin, on the glans penis and/or wherever it hurts. It offers sufferers fast relief by soothing the inflamed areas and easing the intolerable itching and soreness associated with thrush. Pessaries have to be inserted high into the vagina, preferably at night. These melt fairly rapidly. The potent drugs they contain start to kill off all the fungi with which they come into contact. The number of pessaries needed to clear up a fungal infection varies according to the brand being used. Skin disorders of most kinds are difficult to treat. Using too many potent drugs can lower the skin's natural resistance to infection quite dramatically so that the condition easily flares up again. Most doctors prefer short courses of treatment for thrush victims, lasting from three to six days.

There are several kinds of pessaries that can be used to treat thrush. Of these, Canesten, Femeron (Gyno-Daktarin), Pevaryl,

Gyno-Pevaryl, and Ecostatin appear to work best. They are normally used in conjunction with an antifungal cream, such as Canesten, Daktarin or Femeron. Containing broad-spectrum antifungal drugs, they can relieve thrush symptoms in a few hours, though you are not likely to be completely thrush-free for at least two days. No pessary will offer much protection against recurrent thrush and the last three types on this list have an unpleasant side-effect. The drug upon which they are based — econazole — can sometimes irritate the skin rather than soothe it. As the pessaries melt, they begin to sting. This stinging can often be so intense that the sufferer finds it difficult to tell whether it is the thrush or the pessaries that are causing the pain. Econazole, in the form of vaginal pessaries or cream, should never be used during the first three months of pregnancy.

Canesten and Femeron cream and pessaries are now available without prescription, so you can buy them at a chemist's. Daktarin cream can be bought over the counter, too. This is great news for sufferers — you no longer have to wait for a doctor's appointment because, as long as your local chemist is open, you can start treating your thrush immediately! Two courses of Canesten are on sale: a single dose or a pack of three pessaries. Femeron is sold as a single, soft pessary. It is actually exactly the same pessary as a Gyno-Daktarin one, but they are marketed under two different names because the latter brand is targeted at doctors (it is only available on prescription). The manufacturers recommend that it is used overnight. Always remember to read the instructions carefully before use.

Nystatin (Nystan) is an antibiotic that is active against a wide range of fungi and yeast. In the form of powders, drops, ointments, pessaries and tablets (which are taken by mouth), it is used to treat thrush. Longer courses of Nystan pessaries are needed to cure a thrush attack. These may last anything from one week to one month, which is why most sufferers feel unhappy about using them. Keeping to a strict anti-thrush routine for two weeks — no jeans, no tights, no swimming and so on — and having to abstain from sexual contact during this time is all very trying. To go a whole month like this, only to see the infection flare up again once the treatment stops is extremely upsetting. Nystan has another disadvantage in that it is an unpleasant yellow colour. The cream and pessaries will stain your underwear. If you have to use Nystan, for any length of time, pant liners will help to prevent your undies from being ruined.

Vaginal gels

In cases where pessaries of the type mentioned above have failed, some doctors have found that persistent thrush will respond to vaginal gels. These have to be inserted deep into the vagina with a special applicator. Betadine is one such gel. Based on iodine, it is a dark brown/red in colour so that, unfortunately, it will stain your pants. Like Nystan, it has to be taken for long periods of time. This can be a disadvantage but, as most thrust sufferers will agree, any treatment is worth considering while there is still hope of an effective cure.

Oral tablets

Oral tablets are by far the most convenient way to treat thrush — research has shown that women prefer taking an oral treatment rather than mess about with pessaries and creams. Thrush in the bowel or the intestine is almost always the cause of recurrent attacks, and it has been proved that patients with recurrent vaginal thrush are more likely to be cured when they are treated at the same time for intestinal candidiasis.

Essentially, if you have vaginal thrush, it is almost certain that other areas of your body will be infected too, though you may not realize it. So it may be better to take an oral treatment straight off rather than use vaginal pessaries. Diflucan is a one-hit oral thrush treatment and it is now available over the counter (although it is considerably cheaper to 'buy' on prescription if your GP will prescribe it for you — about half the price with current UK charges!). Diflucan is a one-off dose so it's very convenient to take and claims to clear thrush in about three days. One of the main reasons women find recurrent thrush so difficult to cope with is that pessaries are messy and inconvenient to use. One discharge — the one that is associated with thrush — is replaced by another, the leakage from pessaries. In this respect oral tablets have a distinct advantage. Like all oral medications however, they can have side-effects. Reported adverse effects of these types of drugs include nausea, stomach upsets and heartburn, headaches and dizziness. If you are pregnant or breastfeeding, or have a history of medical problems, you must consult your GP before taking Diflucan.

Other tablets such as Nystan, Nizoral and Sporanox are available on prescription.

> I've been suffering from bouts of thrush for the last 18 months, which coincided with my going on the Pill. I was given Canesten pessaries and cream. During a four-month break from the Pill, I still suffered several bouts of thrush. After changing to a female doctor, I was treated in the same way, but eventually she prescribed an oral antifungal called Nizoral. This caused the unpleasant side-effect of diarrhoea, but, since taking a seven-day course six weeks ago, I have not suffered any further attacks.

> I've only had thrush once — touch wood — and that was after a course of antibiotics. My GP prescribed a capsule called Diflucan. I took it and within three days all my symptoms had gone. It was so easy!

If your doctor prescribes an oral treatment for your attack of thrush, always ask for advice on when the tablets should be taken. Sporanax, for example, is most effective if it is taken immediately after a meal.

> I went along to my GP who prescribed Nystan cream, which controls the itching, and new tablets called Nizoral. The tablets have been out about a year. The course lasts for five days or so — two tablets a day, to be taken with food. This was a tip the dispensing chemist gave me. Otherwise, she said, they don't work, because the acid secreted during digestion is necessary for them to be effective.

If you don't want to take oral medication (pregnant women or women trying to conceive should definitely avoid these treatments), eating lost of plain, live yogurt will help to balance your body's flora. Chapter 7 explains more about healing yourself through diet. Attention to your eating habits could mean the difference between your thrush returning a few days or weeks later and not returning at all!

Medicated powders

Thrush is also treated with medicated powders, such as Nystan or

Mycil. In general, powder is more beneficial for men. Its drying effect helps to relieve the inflamed skin. Women can use powder around the vulva, although it should not be applied inside the vagina. Antifungal powders are quite pleasant to use. A frequent dusting down in the genital area would seem an ideal way of helping to prevent recurrent bouts of thrush. By regularly using an antifungal powder, men can play a positive role in helping to rid women of recurrent thrush problems.

Gentian violet

Painting the vagina and cervix with gentian violent is an old-fashioned remedy still used by doctors to treat women prone to vaginal infections like thrush. It can sometimes be effective, but it can also be dangerous and is *not* recommended. Never treat yourself at home with Gentian violet. One woman who accidentally splashed some of the dye into her urethra soon developed severe cystitis. Her bladder became ulcerated and inflamed and she needed urgent hospital treatment. Be warned!

Aci-jel

Aci-jel is called a 'therapeutic vaginal jelly'. It can be bought from chemists and it works in exactly the same way – by making the vagina less favourable to thrush. It is best used as a preventative measure against thrush.

> I have suffered from thrush, on and off, for over a year now. The first time I saw a doctor he prescribed a bottle of Nystatin pills and some Nystatin cream. The cream was useless and the pills were only effective while I was taking them. The second time I went I saw a female doctor . . . She explained the cause and, after a long discussion, she prescribed a therapeutic vaginal gel. This treatment is a bit more successful, although the method of application sometimes puts me off using it.

Cryosurgery

Cryosurgery can also be regarded as a 'cure' for thrush. As mentioned in Chapter 3, many thrush problems are related to cervical irritation. Once an eversion has become troublesome, it becomes more difficult to clear up thrush and other infections present in the vagina. Treating an eversion with cautery or cryosurgery will reduce the likelihood of further attacks of thrush.

Treating oral thrush

Patients suffering from thrush in the mouth are usually prescribed Nystatin liquid or pastilles. Tests show that a week's course of either treatment works equally well, but the general consensus is that the pastilles taste better! Both treatments are more effective if you do not eat or drink for one hour after using them.

Alternatively, you can buy a sugar-free, orange-flavoured gel called Daktarin from your chemist — it is available without prescription, but not advised for women who are or might be pregnant. The gel must be applied four times a day, that is after each meal and before bed. Again, the longer it is left in contact with the infected areas, the better the treatment will work. Daktarin Oral Gel should be continued for at least two days after the symptoms have cleared up.

Oral thrush sufferers can help prevent further attacks by staying fit and healthy, eating a well-balanced diet and avoiding sugary foods and sweets. Smokers suffering from thrush should definitely think about giving up. Sufferers who wear dentures should rigorously sterilize their dentures every day. Asthma sufferers who use a steroid inhaler should rinse the mouth and throat with water after use. Lastly, and possibly most importantly, anyone suffering from oral thrush should aim to treat their whole body, not just the symptoms in their mouth.

Problems with prescribed treatments

Although thrush has a strong tendency to return, for some people, the first attack may well be their last. For many others, though, thrush can recur again and again, lasting for several months at a time. Men and women who are less fortunate have found themselves burdened with a recurrent thrush problem for years.

As it is now believed that recurrent attacks are simply symptoms of overgrowth of *Candida* throughout the whole body, it stands to reason that the root cause must be treated. This is why, of all the treatments mentioned here, oral tablets are the most likely to provide a lasting cure for thrush. This is useful knowledge to have up your sleeve when you walk into your GP's surgery. Many doctors still think the proper cure for thrush is to treat the site of the irritation with creams and pessaries. You might well have to ask for oral tablets yourself, but do not be afraid to speak up!

If, for some reason, you are reluctant to take any tablets by mouth, you can rest assured that other remedies outlined in this chapter are nearly all capable of clearing up an attack of thrush once it has taken hold. In this instance, self-help will prevent further infections developing. The next two chapters in this book are crucial in curing recurrent thrush. Read on!

6
Self-help remedies

Self-help remedies are an alternative to a doctor's powerful drugs. There are lots of different remedies that can be used at home to cure and prevent attacks of thrush, and most of these can be found in the food cupboard. Yogurt, vinegar, and many different types of herbs have been used by women for centuries to treat vaginal infections. Self-help works on the principle that you first restore the vagina's natural ecology, allowing the body to beat the infection and heal itself.

Home remedies may be particularly valuable to the sufferer of *recurrent* thrush and other vaginal infections. Where conventional medicines have failed, it may be that natural therapy will succeed. Obviously not all of the solutions described here will work for everyone. What will work for one woman at one time may be ineffective for that same woman on another occasion. However, self-help remedies are easy to use, cheap and have little or no side-effects. While they may not do any good, they cannot, on the other hand, make the problem any worse, and all of them are worth giving a try.

Most of the remedies described here are liquid solutions. Introducing them into the vagina, and getting them to stay there, presents a tricky problem. Here are some methods that you could try:

- put the solution into the vagina using a spermicide applicator or in a cap
- dampen cotton wool balls in the solution and insert them into the vagina in a cap
- dip or soak a tampon in the mixture/solution, insert into the vagina and leave in place overnight
- place a soaked tampon in a cap, fold it together, and insert it as usual.

Some of the remedies mentioned in this chapter can be poured into a shallowly filled bath. Sit in the bath with your knees apart. Open your vagina by gently inserting a finger or two, pulling down slightly to allow the water to run in.

Yogurt

Yogurt is one of the oldest known and most effective treatments for yeast infections like thrush. It works because it contains cultures of *lactobacilli*, a type of bacteria naturally present throughout the body. In the vagina it plays an important part in keeping *Candida* and other organisms under control. *Lactobacilli* breaks down the glycogen content in the vaginal secretions, converting it into lactic acid. This process keeps the vagina fairly acidic so that potentially harmful bacteria like thrush, which thrive best in alkalinic environments, die. Vaginal infections occur when this delicate acid/alkaline balance is disturbed. Thrush, for instance, indicates that the vagina is too alkaline. *Lactobacilli* cultures can restore the natural acidity of the vagina and so promote healing.

Plain, unpasteurized yogurt is the best source of *lactobacilli*. Only natural yogurt, with a live *acidophilus* culture, and not the flavoured, fruity variety, will be effective.

To combat fungal infection, yogurt should both be eaten and applied directly to the vagina and perineum (or used in a solution). Attacking the problem from both ends lessens the likelihood of reinfection as the fungus that causes thrush can develop and grow in the intestine. An attack of vaginal thrush may indicate that the fungus is present in the intestine, too. This can be corrected within a few days by eating lots of yogurt or *acidophilus* milk or culture.

In all cases, yogurt should be used at the first signs of infection. Use natural yogurt (live) directly, inserting it into the vagina twice a day for about a week. Rubbing plain yogurt on the irritated skin around the vagina will help to soothe the inflammation.

To make a yogurt solution, add about two or three tablespoons of plain yogurt to 1.2 litres (2 pints) of warm water. Use daily for up to a week. Alternatively, buy *acidophilus* culture from a healthfood shop. This contains a *lactobacilli* culture in liquid form. Use this twice a day for one week. *Acidophilus* capsules can be bought from healthfood shops. Insert one into the vagina twice a day for one week.

Many women find that by using yogurt at the first signs of infection, an attack of thrush can be relieved within hours. Usually it will disappear after only a few days of treatment. If, however, the symptoms still persist after a week, it is best to stop treating it yourself and to visit a doctor.

After having thrush on and off for two years, I solved my problem by changing from the Pill to the cap and using yogurt to treat the residual infection, having had no joy with Nystan pessaries. This I applied either in my cap or with tampons for about ten days. (I used, of course, natural yogurt.) I've finally got rid of thrush.

I, too, was a sufferer — intermittently for about four years, significantly, while I was on the Pill. I was treated with antibiotic pessaries when I eventually plucked up courage to seek treatment, but wasn't happy about it. A young female GP suggested an old-fashioned remedy — *natural yogurt*! Instant success and relief within a few hours — if a trifle messy!

Tea tree oil

Australian tea tree oil (*melaleuca alternifolia*) has been around for centuries. The Aboriginal people knew of its healing qualities, treating their cuts and wounds with the crushed leaves of the tea trees growing around their creeks. During the Second World War, tea tree oil was included in the Army's kits in the South Pacific to treat fungal infections such as foot rot.

It is often called a miracle oil because it is non-toxic, non-irritant and a stronger germicide than carbolic. Tea tree essential oil — a pure and powerful extract from the plant — is both antiseptic and antifungal. Australians refer to it as the first aid kit in a bottle! Whatever, tea tree oil is an extremely effective weapon in the war against thrush. It is available from all good healthfood shops and can be used in a number of different ways.

- *As a bath oil* Add a few drops to your bath water.
- *Use directly* Because it is virtually non-irritant, even to the most sensitive tissues, you can use tea tree oil directly on your skin, but do not overdo it. All essential oils should be used sparingly because they are so powerful. Put *one* drop of tea tree oil on a cotton bud. Use this to swab around the vagina and/or infected areas.
- *Pessaries and creams* These are available by post from the House of Mistry, (see page 115 for their address) and are sold in boxes of six, but you might find their products in large healthfood shops. It is suggested that one is used at night, but, if symptoms persist,

visit your doctor. House of Mistry enjoy a lot of very positive feedback from their customers and claim that 'they are effective and gentle in treating thrush'.

> I suffered from recurrent thrush on and off for about a year. My doctor prescribed pessaries but these were only effective for a short while. When my period returned, so did my thrush. I read about tea tree oil in a magazine and decided to try some out. I added a few drops to my bath and on the last days of my period I'd put a few drops of the oil on my tampons. It worked! I haven't had an attack for nine months. And when I do feel a bit twingey, I nip an attack in the bud with my *essential* essential oil!

Tea tree oil has also been shown to cure boils, athlete's foot, and acne among other things. Gargling with warm water and a drop of the oil can stave off a throat infection. Like other essential oils, tea tree oil stimulates the immune system, so, if used at the earliest opportunity, it will help the body to fight an infection itself.

Vinegar

Vinegar and, to an extent, lemon juice, help to restore the acid balance of the vagina. Using weak solutions of vinegar and lemon juice can sometimes cure an attack of thrush. Vinegar and salt solutions are also helpful in treating non-specific vaginal infections.

Use about two tablespoons of white, sugarless vinegar or lemon juice to 600 ml (1 pint) of water. Soak a tampon in this solution and then insert into the vagina overnight. You could try pouring a little vinegar into a shallowly filled bath and sitting down in it for about five minutes, but remember that long soaks in hot water can do more harm than good.

Salt is a neutralizing agent. Salt baths are therapeutic as they help to soothe and heal inflamed mucous membranes. For a non-specific infection, alternate vinegar and salt water solutions for a week — use the vinegar solution one day, the salt water solution the next and so on. Add about half a tablespoon of salt (or two tablespoons of vinegar) to every 600 ml (1 pint) of water that you use.

Bicarbonate of soda

Some women have found relief from thrush with bicarbonate of soda, either in the form of sodamints (indigestion tablets) inserted high into the vagina, or simply by diluting the bicarbonate in their bathwater. Treating thrush in this way is slightly unusual. Other cures work by making the vagina more acidic — too acidic for *Candida* to grow in. Bicarbonate of soda is used to increase the vagina's alkalinity so that it is too alkaline even for the fungi to survive.

Sodamints are difficult to obtain as they have gone out of fashion in recent years. Some chemists may still stock them, however, and certain pharmacists may be prepared to make them up for you. Certain healthfood shops may also be able to help. Otherwise, add a little bicarbonate of soda to the bathwater, or use with a mild solution of bicarbonate of soda and cool water.

Garlic

Garlic is well known for its healing properties. It is a form of antibiotic and has been used for centuries by women to treat vaginal infections.

Like tea tree oil, garlic is extremely powerful against yeasts and fungi as well as bacteria. A recent report proved garlic to be more active against human ringworm (a fungal infection) than currently prescribed drug treatments.

Garlic is useful when more than one infection is present in the vagina at any one time.

- Put eight cloves of garlic in a jar with about 300 ml (½ pint) of white, sugarless vinegar. Leave this by a window for about two days, until the oil of the garlic has been released. Use a tablespoon of this solution in 600 ml (1 pint) of water. Use twice a day for a week.
- If an irritation develops, then just use a garlic solution. Simply boil 600 ml (1 pint) of water and add a peeled and chopped clove of garlic. Boil together for about 15 minutes, strain and leave to cool. Use twice a day for a week.
- Garlic cloves can be inserted into the vagina, and perhaps in this way, work more effectively. Slice a clove in half. Wrap it in gauze. Insert into the vagina and leave overnight.

Spermicides

Spermicidal jellies and foams are a useful form of contraceptive when they are used correctly in conjunction with a condom or cap. They *may* protect women against some sexually transmitted diseases like gonorrhoea, and *may* offer protection against cancer of the cervix. They *may* also help to prevent vaginal infections like thrush. It is possible that they inhibit bacterial and fungal growth. They can be bought from any chemist and used as a preventative measure against thrush. Some women, however, develop an allergic reaction to spermicides (see Chapter 9), and they can actually be the source of a vaginal infection.

Herbs

Here are some simple herbal remedies that are effective in curing and preventing thrush. Like most self-help remedies, they work by restoring the body to its normal state and, again, are inexpensive. Herbal solutions can be inserted into the vagina. It is also possible to make poultices (herb-soaked pads) that help to relieve the external itching and soreness associated with thrush, while they fight the infection inside.

You can use fresh or dried herbs. Buying in bulk is cheaper. To prepare a herbal solution, boil the specified amount of herb (usually 10–25 g (½–1 oz)) in about 1.2 litres (2 pints) of water. Strain the liquid and always allow it to cool before use. Never use aluminium utensils to prepare herbs.

Herbal solutions

Bayberry Bark

Boil 1.2 litres (2 pints) of water. Add two to three tablespoons of bayberry bark, and boil gently for about 20 minutes. Strain the liquid and leave to cool. Use daily for a week.

Goldenseal and myrrh

Boil 900 ml (1½ pints) of water. Add a tablespoon of goldenseal and one tablespoon of myrrh. Simmer for 20 minutes. Strain the liquid. Use daily for a week to treat thrush and/or *Trichomonas* (see Chapter 8).

Goldenseal is also good for any vaginitis. Boil 600 ml (1 pint) of water. Add one teaspoon of goldenseal powder. Simmer for 20–30 minutes. Add enough water to make up 1.2 litres (2 pints) in total. Use daily for one week.

Thuja

Thuja is an antifungal herb. It is available as an ointment from healthfood shops and herbalists. This can be smeared on to a tampon or added to water to make a solution. Ten drops of thuja diluted in a glass of water can also be drunk three times daily.

Calendula (marigold), slippery elm, black willow bark, pit root and fennel seed, rosemary and sage can be used to treat all non-specific vaginitis. Chickweed, chaparral and chamomile are effective in treating *Trichomonas*.

Herbal poultices

Herb-soaked pads can be held to the genital area for five minutes to several hours to relieve external itching. To make a herbal poultice, use fresh herbs wrapped in muslin or cotton. Dampen the pad slightly, and change when it becomes dry.

Cottage cheese

Cottage cheese, wrapped in muslin and worn on a sanitary towel daily for two weeks can be helpful in treating thrush. The cheese relieves the itching and soreness associated with thrush and apparently helps to draw the infection out of the system. This poultice should be changed several times a day, according to the severity of the attack. It is reported to be most effective when oatstraw tea is drunk daily.

Oatstraw tea

Add one teaspoon to one cup of boiling water. Drink daily for a month while you are being treated for a fungal infection. A stronger tea, allowed to steep for 15 minutes, can be used as a poultice or added to the bathwater.

Aromatherapy

Aromatherapy is a mixture of aromas, massage and medicine, and uses essential oils extracted from plants, flowers, bushes and herbs. Our sense of smell is so closely linked to our emotions that it is not hard to recognize the power of aromatherapy. Also, massage relaxes and soothes the body by relieving tension and encouraging the release of pent-up emotions. Massage can also increase your 'feel-good factor'. This is because it stimulates the release of hormones known as *endorphins*. These act as natural painkillers, relaxants and euphoriants. Importantly, too, massage can enhance your body's own healing potential.

In her book, *Aromatherapy for Women*, Maggie Tisserand recommends several essential oil treatments for thrush sufferers. These are listed below and may work well for some women.

Internal medication for Candida

Take three drops niaouli, three drops lemon on half a teaspoon of brown sugar. The dosage can be repeated twice per day for a maximum of three weeks. If any stomach upset follows, Maggie recommends reducing the amount of oil drops to one niaouli and one lemon, or stopping taking the treatment until your stomach feels fine again.

Bath solution

Add tea tree, rose and lavender oils to your bath.

Vaginal pessary

Drop tea tree oil across the top and sides of a tampon and insert it into the vagina. This is best done overnight.

Aloe vera

Aloe vera extract is known for its healing properties. Pure aloe vera juice diluted, dabbed on cotton wool and swabbed over the most itchy areas is said to soothe thrush. A little aloe vera oil on a tampon may be effective, too. Aloe vera mouthwash will help oral thrush.

Some other points

Natural remedies can be very potent. If one is going to work for you, it will have done so within a week. Unless otherwise directed, it is best to use these treatments at the *first* signs of an infection and to continue to do so for the next seven days. If after this time you still think you have an infection, it is worth reassessing your problem. Perhaps it is time to consult your doctor.

Although thrush is not a serious disease, it is important to treat it at its first signs. The symptoms of thrush are such that they can easily be confused with other infections. Vaginal discharge, irritation and soreness could indicate a multitude of infections from non-specific vaginitis through to more serious diseases like gonorrhoea. Similarly two or more infections may also be present in the vagina alongside thrush. They need to be properly diagnosed and appropriately treated.

7
Diet

> I have been plagued with thrush for the last six months, but was not aware then what it was. I did not approach a doctor until the itching made me totally miserable. I was treated with a vaginal cream, but it never actually cleared up. I was still having a discharge and itching and was particularly worse on days after I'd eaten nothing but sweet things and not a proper meal.

Of all the information about self-help measures that we can take to protect ourselves against thrush, dietary advice seems to be the hardest to obtain. Diet plays a vital role in helping to safeguard the body against illness and yet how many of us have ever been warned that the foods we eat — or are not eating, as the case may be — are contributing to a recurrent thrush problem?

A sensible diet should keep us in good health. An attack of thrush is often a sign of poor eating habits. By reassessing the value of the things we eat, we can take a positive step forward in helping ourselves to better health.

What is a healthy diet? Food is needed for energy and for the growth and maintenance of the human body. Protein, fat and carbohydrate are the three basic nutrients that can provide this energy. All foods contain various amounts of proteins, fats and/or carbohydrates. Some foods are high in vitamins and minerals that are essential for good health. They help to prevent disease and keep our blood and tissue fluid functioning. They keep our skin and our hair in good condition, and much more besides.

A healthy diet must be a balanced diet. It should contain all of the nutrients our body needs — proteins, fats, carbohydrates, vitamins and minerals. A diet that lacks one or more of these requirements may have quite serious short-term or long-term effects. For example, carbohydrates are very important because they assist in the assimilation and digestion of other foods. Fat and carbohydrate (sugar) are both sources of energy, but fat cannot easily be burnt off without the presence of sugar. Protein is primarily a body 'builder'. It is utilized by the body to repair and build up the skin, the hair, the muscles and all of our internal organs, too. When we eat less fat and carbohydrate, protein has to be used to provide energy, though it may be badly needed for repairing and replacing damaged cells within the body.

People in the Western world today eat a large proportion of refined or processed foods. These have little of the nutritional content of fresh, untreated foods. Valuable vitamins and minerals are lost during the refining process. Also, convenience foods lack the roughage or fibre that the body needs to get rid of its waste products.

Refined sugar has become an accepted part of our lives. We eat too much of it. We take it in our tea and coffee, in soft drinks like cola and lemonade, and in cakes, sweets and chocolate bars. We have developed a 'sweet tooth' and, consequently, our health suffers.

An excessive amount of sugar in the diet can be dangerous for several reasons: it interferes with the absorption of proteins, calcium and many other minerals, it destroys the valuable bacteria that live in our intestines which help to keep us healthy, too much sugar overstimulates the production of insulin and can cause diabetes, and sugar is the great aggravator of thrush.

The connection between sugar and thrush

The mucous membranes of the vaginal walls secrete glycogen, a sugar compound. Bacteria that live in the vagina, called *lactobacilli*, ferment this sugar into lactic acid. This process inhibits fungal growth and keeps vaginal infections at bay. It maintains the pH balance of the vagina at just the right level, so that it is too acidic for thrush and other organisms to survive in.

The intestines are populated by the same sort of *bacilli*. They are invaluable there. They, too, feed on sugar and produce lactic acid to destroy potentially harmful organisms fighting for survival in the gut. Similar bacteria are present in the mouth, working to the same ends. They break down sugar, forming lactic acid in the process. It is this acid that causes tooth decay — another reason for avoiding sugar and sweets!

Eating large quantities of sugar has a negative effect on our intestinal, vaginal and oral bacteria. *Lactobacilli* are unable to cope with the amount of sugar in the intestinal tract. They cannot ferment all the sugar into lactic acid. They cannot suppress the disease — and odour-producing bacteria that surround them. Once the 'bad' organisms gain a hold in the body, they multiply out of all proportion, using the sugar to their advantage — fungi thrive on sugar.

An abundance of thrush in the gut and bowel will soon infect the vagina. A general absence of 'good' bacteria throughout the body stimulates the growth of thrush anywhere — in the mouth, in the stomach, in the bowel and in the vagina. This is the connection between sugar and thrush. Sugar not only destroys beneficial organisms in the body; it also encourages degenerative bacteria to grow. Recurring thrush may be caused by a high carbohydrate intake.

Carbohydrates

There are many sources of sugar in the diet. All of these sources are classed as *carbohydrates*; a group of foods that contain sugar, starch and/or cellulose. During digestion, all starch is converted into sugar, and all sugar is then broken down into glucose. In this form, starches and sugars can be absorbed into the bloodstream. Some glucose is used in the tissues to provide energy wherever it is required. The remainder is recombined to form glycogen. This can be stored in the liver and muscles until it is needed. As the level of glucose in the blood begins to fall, glycogen stores are released and broken down again. The level of glucose in the bloodstream is carefully regulated by this process.

Although all carbohydrate foods are eventually converted into sugar, there are certain foods in this group that are 'better' than others. These are called *superior carbohydrates*. They are supplied by root vegetables, wholegrain breads and cereals, and fresh fruits. They are 'better' because in these foods the conversion of starch into sugar is gradual. Sugar is released slowly, in quantities that the intestinal bacteria can manage.

Superior carbohydrates are particularly high in vitamins and minerals, and in cellulose. Cellulose has little energy value, but provides fibre to help the body eliminate its waste products. These foods, in modest amounts, are valuable and necessary in our diet, and there is no reason why they should be avoided.

If you suffer from recurrent thrush, you should cut down your intake of *refined* foods. These tend to be the worst carbohydrate source. They contain little or no fibre. The amount of vitamins and minerals they supply is greatly reduced during the refining process. Many women find that an attack of thrush occurs after they have been over-indulging in sweets, cakes and biscuits.

Without eating refined sugar in any form, a combination of natural sugars and sugar-formers, together with the sugar freed during the digestion of starch, brings our total sugar intake up to a surprisingly large amount. When we eat foods of a high carbohydrate content we can consume more than 450 g (1 lb) of sugar a day, and this does not even take into account the sugar we might heap into our hot drinks or on to our morning cereal as well! Other foodstuffs are deceptively high in sugar: baked beans, bananas, figs, macaroni, noodles, plums and prunes, and, particularly, tinned and dried fruits.

By eating sensibly, we can help our bodies to fight infection, and we can prevent recurrences of vaginal thrush. Always be wary of refined sugars, flours, cereals and breads. In effect, this means avoiding most of the things we love to eat — chocolate, cakes, sweet sauces, jams and marmalades. White bread, rolls and buns, and white flour, packaged cereals, rice and pasta should be replaced with brown, wholegrain foods.

To keep thrush at bay, and to keep healthy, choose your carbohydrate intake from those foods that have an unusually low sugar content: asparagus, beetroots, Brussels sprouts, cabbage, carrots, cauliflower, celery, cucumbers, kale, leeks, lettuce, dried onions, green peppers, pumpkin, radishes, rhubarb, spinach, string beans, tomatoes and watercress. These foods are also low in calories and contain lots of vitamins and minerals.

Diabetes

Diabetic women are highly susceptible to thrush, owing to the fact that they have high or uncontrolled levels of sugar in their blood. Diabetes means that the body is unable to break down and use its foods properly. This is because diabetics are either deficient in insulin — a hormone secreted by the pancreas — or because their bodies do not react properly to the insulin they produce. Insulin makes it possible for sugar (glucose) to enter the cells to be converted into energy. As this sugar can neither enter the cells nor be utilized as energy, it accumulates in the bloodstream. When the glucose level gets too high, sugar spills into the urine. The kidneys have to provide more urine to carry this glucose. The body needs to replace the excessive amounts of urine that the diabetic produces. Severe thirst and an increased need to urinate are the earliest symptoms of the disease.

Women with diabetes have extra sugar in their vaginal walls and this encourages the growth of thrush. Sugar in the urine, deposited on the vulva, provides food for the fungus. Undetected diabetes may be the source of a recurrent thrush problem. Unless the diabetes is brought under control it is very likely that the thrush will continue to be a problem.

Diabetes can be treated. Some patients will need a daily injection of insulin. In cases where the diabetic is capable of producing insulin but only in small amounts, they will need to reduce their carbohydrate intake to a quantity that their own insulin supplies can deal with.

If you are persistently plagued with thrush, it is important that you be tested for diabetes, especially if there is a history of the disease in your family. The presence of sugar in the urine can indicate diabetes, but your doctor should refer you to a hospital for a *full glucose tolerance test.* You will be asked not to eat or drink anything for at least eight hours before the test, which takes about two and a half hours. It is a good idea to take something to read along with you to help to pass the time, and a small snack to eat afterwards. During the test you will be given drinks of glucose. After each drink a sample of your blood will be taken to check the level of glucose. You will be asked for a urine sample before and on completion of the test.

The results of a full glucose tolerance test should come through in about a week. If they are negative and you do not have diabetes, the cause of thrush must lie elsewhere.

Vital vitamins

Vitamins are vital for good health. They are essential for healthy growth and development. If a diet is lacking in one or more of these nutrients, your body will suffer. For example, vitamin C (ascorbic acid) is vital in building up the body's resistance to disease. It also helps prevent allergies. Cabbages, tomatoes and citrus fruits are the richest sources of vitamin C, but it is found in all fresh fruits and vegetables.

A link has been made between *Candida* and certain vitamin deficiencies. These include vitamin A (retinol), found mainly in liver, butter and green and orange vegetables, which helps to keep the mucous membranes in good condition. Vitamin A is fat-soluble. It can be stored in the body, unlike vitamin C, which must be supplied daily.

Chapters 2 and 3 dealt with the sort of things that encourage the growth of *Candida*. Some of these should now be discussed again. The Pill, sugar, diabetes and antibiotics are all relevant here. Why? Because of the link between them and vitamin B_6. All of these things increase the body's need for this particular vitamin. The Pill and antibiotics, diabetes and an excessive intake of sugar can cause a deficiency of vitamin B_6, and all of them lower the body's resistance to fungal infection. This strongly suggests, therefore, that vitamin B_6 is one of the keys to preventing thrush. It is worth noting here that vitamin B_6 is also recommended as a cure for PMT. You may recall my mentioning earlier that PMT may well be just a side-effect of *Candida*. This is why vitamin B_6, which can help prevent thrush, will also effectively treat PMT.

> I was desperate. I tried everything that people advised, but the most effective way was my increase in vitamin B_6 (pyridoxine). I take 100 milligrams per day and there is no worry of 'overdosing' as they are water-soluble. They will be flushed out of the body if not used. As all my efforts with external applications did not work, I thought that attacking the thrush internally would be successful. I have increased my total intake of the B vitamins.

The vitamin B family, or vitamin B complex as it is known, consists of about 18 different members. Of these at least 12 can be made chemically. Most of these vitamins are obtained from the same sources so that an inadequate diet will usually be deficient in several of the B vitamins rather than just one of them. Brewer's yeast, wheatgerm and meat are rich in all of the B vitamins. Nuts, beans and lentils, and soya products are other good sources.

Vitamin B_1 (thiamin), essential for growth, the conversion of carbohydrates into energy, and the health of the nerves and muscles, is found in most wholegrain foods. Seafood also contains small amounts. Vitamin B_2 (riboflavin), which helps to keep the skin, mouth and eyes healthy, is supplied in eggs, vegetables, milk and cheese. Vitamin B_6 (pyridoxine) can be obtained from most wholemeal products, oats, milk, fish and cabbage. Liver, meat and eggs provide supplies of vitamin B_{12} (cyanocobalamine). Choline and insotitol are essential for the functioning of the liver and to prevent the build-up of fats in the body. Folic acid is used for making red blood cells. These substances are supplied by offal meats, nuts, green vegetables, yeast and wheatgerm.

A lack of the B vitamins is mainly caused by eating too many refined foods, or overcooking fresh sources of the vitamins. Like vitamin C, they are all water-soluble. They dissolve in water just as sugar or salt does. This means that they are easily lost by cooking foods in water, and they cannot be stored in the body. (Vitamin B_{12} is an exception. It can be stored in the liver.) If they are not used, any excess will be passed out of the body in the urine. To keep healthy, make sure you get a good intake of the B vitamins every day.

A deficiency of vitamin B complex affects the nerves and may result in nervous disorders and depression. These may be indirect causes of thrush. A lack of the B vitamins can also result in diseases of the skin, and what is thrush if it is not a skin disease? During illness, a person's need for vitamin B increases. A vitamin B deficiency makes you prone to thrush, which is why we get attacks when we are poorly, under stress or generally run down.

If you eat too much sugar, you are more likely to develop thrush. Women on the Pill who eat large amounts of carbohydrate may be suffering from attacks, not simply because the fungus thrives on sugar, but also because they are deficient in vitamin B_6. A high sugar intake destroys the good *bacilli* in the intestine and can cause diabetes. Because the B vitamins are water-soluble, they are readily lost in the urine. Diabetics who excrete large amounts of urine are usually lacking in these vitamins, especially vitamin B_6. This is yet another reason for them being so defenceless against thrush.

Certain intestinal bacteria are capable of synthesizing the B vitamins, so, even if your intake of foods containing vitamin B is low, the body may still be producing enough to protect you from thrush. However, when these bacteria are destroyed, by antibiotics, for example, or by eating too much sugar, a higher intake of vitamin B will be necessary to prevent fungal growth.

Thrush can be kept at bay by cutting down on sugar *and* increasing your intake of vitamin B. On average, we require at least three milligrams of vitamin B_1, and from three to five milligrams of vitamin B_2 daily. During an attack, eat plenty of those foods rich in the B vitamins. Obtain the optimum amount of vitamin B complex as a safeguard against further infections.

> I have been a 'lifelonger'. Thrush ebbs and flows with my general state of health, but is ever lurking. I once had a long talk with a very understanding (lady) doctor. She seemed to think my

> lifelong eczema was related to the thrush, especially when I mentioned that I'd been fed copious quantities of vitamin B as a child, and still seemed to need it. She recommended taking vitamin B, either naturally or in concentrated pill form and it does seem to help enormously. It also seems to help PMT, something I was suffering from more and more as I got older.

Vitamin B tablets are no real substitute for proper vitamin B-rich foods, and if you eat plenty of food containing vitamin B, you will not need to take supplementary tablets. Extra vitamin B cannot be stored in the body. It will be excreted in the urine. However, if you are not getting your maximum quota of vitamin B through your diet, it is advisable to take a supplementary dosage in tablet form. These can be bought from most healthfood shops and chemists.

Yogurt

Eating *acidophilus* culture (found in live yogurt) helps maintain the natural ecology of the *small* intestine. *Bifidobacteria*, also found in live yogurt, does the same job in the *large* intestine. As mentioned before, these bacteria also produce vitamin B. So eating live yogurt is one of the best ways to take vitamin B as it both replaces and restores these bacteria, which, in turn, will produce more of this vitamin. All the B vitamins can be synthesized by the bacteria found in yogurt and/or *acidophilus* culture.

This type of yogurt can be bought from healthfood shops, but home-made yogurt is even better. When made with non-instant powdered milk, it contains twice the amount of protein, calcium and vitamin B_2 that commercially produced yogurt does, and it is cheaper, too!

> I thoroughly recommend natural yogurt — it is good for the gut as it repopulates it with the right gut flora, and good for the genitals as it is incredibly soothing. How many foods are so good for one at both ends?

Making your own yogurt

You will need to buy a tub of live yogurt or *acidophilus* culture before you can make your own.

Heat 1.2 litres (2 pints) of milk in a saucepan. Bring to the boil and leave to cool until it is only slightly warm. Stir the tub of yogurt or *acidophilus* culture into the lukewarm milk. Then pour this into empty cartons, cups or jars and cover. Leave them in a warm place to curdle (this takes about three to six hours). The yogurt must be kept warm so that the bacteria it contains can multiply and sour the milk entirely.

When a thick, firm curd has formed over the milk, the yogurt should be placed in the fridge. This prevents further bacterial growth and stops the milk from becoming too sour. After about eight hours in the refrigerator, the yogurt should be ready to eat.

More can be made using a part of the yogurt from your first batch as a new culture. After a month you will probably need to refresh the yogurt with a more concentrated bought culture.

Minerals

Like vitamins, minerals are essential for keeping disease and ill health at bay. Iron, magnesium and zinc have been pinpointed as beneficial in preventing thrush. Among their numerous functions, they keep the blood and tissue fluids from becoming either too acid or too alkaline. This, of course, is of great importance in controlling thrush.

> I am 41 years old. I have suffered from thrush for about four years. I got so many attacks that seldom a month passed without it. I got so depressed and tearful last November that I went to talk to a lady doctor at my local Well Woman clinic. She explained what a vicious circle it all was and sent me back to my own doctor. This time, however, he said that he and a colleague had a theory that the iron level in the blood had something to do with women being susceptible to thrush. So I have had a long course of iron tablets and have not had an attack for four months now.

Women are more prone to thrush when they become anaemic; that is, when they develop a shortage of haemoglobin. Iron is essential because it combines with protein to form haemoglobin. This is the oxygen-carrying component of the red blood cells. Iron allows the blood to function properly and keeps our tissues healthy. Women are more likely to be deficient in iron than men and, thus, are more susceptible to anaemia. The average human body contains about three or four grams of iron. Some of this will be lost via the outermost layer of skin, which the body continuously sheds. During menstruation, women lose about 30 milligrams each month. In pregnancy, the need for iron increases significantly. Green leafy vegetables, such as broccoli and spinach, are rich in iron, and the vitamin C that they also contain improves the absorption of iron from the intestine. Liver, meat, eggs and cereals are also good sources of this mineral.

Leaky gut syndrome, food allergies and toxemia

Left unchecked, a *Candida* overgrowth in the intestines will cause problems. It can damage the mucus-covered lining there and lead to *leaky gut syndrome*. This is when the walls of the intestine become more permeable; it is easier for molecules to pass through the walls of the intestine. Leaky gut syndrome also makes it easier for the harmful organisms to pass back into the body from the bowel, and, if this happens, the sufferer is more likely to develop a form of toxemia, with symptoms such as headaches, dizziness, fainting and nausea. Patients suffering from *Candida* often complain of feeling bloated or craving carbohydrates.

Leaky gut syndrome also encourages food allergies to develop. This is because the gut allows large molecules of undigested food protein to enter the bloodstream, thus causing an immune reaction. However, allergies may well fade once the thrush has been eliminated, and the damage done to the bowel lining by the excessive *Candida* can be repaired. Fish oils, found in oily fish like mackerel and herring, but available in supplement form, can heal the bowel lining. However, the best way to protect yourself from *Candida* taking a hold in the gut is to stay happy and healthy.

Roughage

The importance of a high-fibre diet cannot be stressed enough. Roughage in a diet avoids constipation by increasing the activity of the muscles in the bowel wall. Diets low in fibre leave the bowel wall with very little to work on. As a result, constipation occurs, leading to stagnation of the bowel's contents. When the contents of the bowel move slowly or stagnate, potentially harmful bacteria can develop there.

Fibre is not easily absorbed through the bowel wall. It passes through the whole length of the bowel, trapping organisms and bacteria within its meshes. In this way, it stops harmful bacteria coming into contact with the bowel walls and breeding there.

Natural, high-fibre foods cleanse the bowel of toxins. A diet high in natural fibre will help you flush thrush away!

Boost your immune system

It is much easier to get thrush when your immunity is low — for example after an illness or if your eating habits are poor — so building up your immune system is essential. One of the best ways to do this is through your diet.

When a person's immune system is weak, a variety of complaints often affect them. Feeling tired all the time or having headaches and being depressed are typical. However, when the immune system is not functioning properly, even more serious disorders may develop, including cancer and acquired immune deficiency syndrome, AIDS, mentioned in Chapter 8.

Environmental chemicals weaken our immune systems, and it is not only industrial and farm chemicals that can be dangerous. Poisons like tobacco, lead from car exhaust fumes and metals such as aluminium and mercury can cause problems, too.

The immune system is part of your body's natural protection against an environment that constantly threatens your well-being. It includes *antibodies* and many different kinds of *white blood cells.* They work like an army, navy and airforce defending the body against enemies. First, they identify what these may be, then they neutralize, conquer or eliminate them!

Your skin is the front line of defence to keep dangers at bay. Mucous membranes line the *interior* cavities and passageways of the body. These membranes act as a barrier against invaders. The mucus coating them contains antibodies to fight infection. Thrush infects the membranes, causing an irritating inflammation and other problems, as we have seen. In doing so, it also weakens the protection these membranes provide against other diseases. It is, therefore, essential to keep these membranes healthy. This can be achieved by eating the right kinds of foods. Boost your immune system with natural nutrients like vitamin C, the oils found in fish, and plenty of iron, magnesium and zinc. It is worth remembering that alcohol and caffeine, found in tea and coffee, stress the immune system.

*The anti-*Candida *diet*

This chapter has specifically dealt with diet. Hopefully you will now know that what we eat contributes enormously to your health and well-being. It is really important now to conclude this chapter by laying down the basis of an anti-*Candida* diet. The following points bring together all that has been said earlier.

Foods to avoid

- *Avoid all fermented drinks* This means alcohol! Alcohol is particularly bad for the body because it contains a lot of sugar and because it increases the body's need for vitamin B_1. It also inflames the mucous membranes. Beer and light wines are less irritant to the body than spirits as their alcohol content is more diluted.
- *Avoid all foods with a high mould content* For example mushrooms and cheese or cheesy snacks. Blue cheeses, such as Roquefort, are the worst. Nuts attract mould so it is wise to give them up, too!
- *Avoid foods with yeast in them* Marmite and yeast extract are not to be taken. Do not take brewers' yeast tablets or vitamin supplements that contain yeasts — if in doubt, check the label.
- *Avoid food additives* Monosodium glutamate, for example, is a yeast derivative. Smoked meats and fish, sausages and hot dogs all contain additives, too, some of which will be derived from yeasts — beware!
- *Avoid all foods containing vinegar — or fermented foodstuffs* This category includes ketchup, mustard, soy sauce, pickles, relishes, salad cream and so on.
- *Avoid refined sugar, dairy produce and artificial sweeteners* One survey linked incidences of thrush and those whose diet included a lot of refined sugar, dairy produce and artificial sweeteners. When these foods were cut out, the number of attacks of thrush, and their severity, were dramatically reduced.
- *Eat fewer eggs and fat-laden dairy products.*

Foods to eat more of

- *Stick to a low-carbohydrate diet* Avoid *all* refined carbohydrates and sugars, and, instead, choose superior carbohydrates, such as potatoes, carrots, asparagus, aubergines and greens.
- *One or two servings of fresh fruit a day* However, some people

who have followed an anti-*Candida* diet have found that fruit makes their problem worse. This could be because fruits are loaded with fructose, a natural sugar. If you find this, too, then avoid fruit at first, then gradually reintroduce it into your diet, after three weeks or so. If you like fruit juice, buy a juicer and make it fresh yourself. It is cheaper and tastes better this way, too! Cartons of fruit juice and fruit drinks often contain *citric acid*, a yeast derivative.

- *Eat lots of yogurt* Although yogurt is fermented, it can actually help cure thrush, so you can eat plenty of it, as long as it is unsweetened and contains live cultures.
- *Eat as much raw garlic as you can* Crush it with oil and lemon juice and use as a salad dressing, or eat it blended with avocado, tomato and onions as a delicious dip. As well as being a powerful antibiotic, garlic can kill yeasts and fungi.
- *Fill yourself up on brown rice instead of bread* Bread is a baked food that has been risen with yeast, so avoid it.
- *Eat oily fish instead of meat*
- *Let vegetables dominate your diet* Eat them raw whenever possible or lightly steamed. A diet high in vegetables such as cabbage, broccoli and cauliflower is believed to offer protection against developing cancer, too.

I started with thrush over four years ago and much to my annoyance still have this. Not only do I ruin my underwear, but the irritation of the itchiness and burning is awful and embarrassing.

I eat plenty of food, and find cheese, coffee and rich food contribute to a certain level of the thrush because, after eating many of these, I find it probably at its worst and the start of it yet again.

To cut a long story short. . . . A couple of years ago, a friend mentioned a lady doctor who sounded sane, sensible and interested in women's complaints. Off I went to see her. She gave me a long list of foods to cut out of my diet. This was after I had done some research on myself by following and listing the results of a three-week rotating diet. It was hard work, but I was determined. Eventually, she had me cut out the following foods: cheese — mould forms on it, mushrooms — a fungus, alcohol — made from fermented fruit, yeasty bread — most breads have

> yeast! I cut them all out and things improved. I have stopped drinking and eating mushrooms and cheese completely. I still have a little bread. Sugar also aggravated the thrush situation for me.

Changing your diet may be *the* change for the better. A thrush problem may be caused or perpetuated by something in your diet. Try not to eat any of the suspect foods like cheese for at least ten days, and see what difference this makes. Should the symptoms of thrush return on resuming your normal diet, it would be wise to avoid these foods permanently. It is possible that your body only reacts to one food in particular. To pinpoint exactly what is causing the trouble, cut out several of the 'baddies' listed in this chapter week by week from your diet. For example, during the first week eliminate sweets and sugary foods. The following week stop eating cheese and so on until the symptoms associated with thrush disappear. If an attack flares up again after an over-indulgence of one of these foods, you will know for certain which one is your enemy!

Making food your medicine need not be unpleasant. Try not to think about the foods that are now crossed off your shopping list. Acquire a taste for, and positively enjoy, nature's gifts that will help you reach the peak of fitness, and remember that good health means good riddance to thrush!

8
About other genital infections

Apart from thrush, there are many other diseases that can affect our sexual and reproductive organs. Most of these are extremely common. Some are caused by bacteria, others are spread by a virus. Some are caught by sexual contact, and these are called *venereal*, or sexually transmitted diseases (STDs). Venereal diseases must be treated immediately as they can become more serious and cause permanent damage to your health and fertility.

All of the conditions described in this chapter can cause severe discomfort and emotional distress, especially when they recur. More importantly, though, the symptoms of so many of these infections can easily be mistaken for thrush. A survey among regular sufferers of thrush revealed that most of them were well able to recognize the symptoms of *Candida*. They were able to diagnose thrush in themselves. As it is no longer necessary to visit a doctor to receive treatment for thrush, it has become more crucial than ever that sufferers know about other infections. If there is the slightest possibility that you might be suffering from one or another of the conditions described in this chapter, visit your doctor as soon as possible.

Trichomonas

This is an infection caused by the parasite, *Trichomonas vaginalis*, a tiny, one-celled organism that feeds on other cells. The organism survives in warm, moist environments. In some women it is a normal and harmless inhabitant of the vagina and bladder. When too many of these bugs are present, an infection will flare up.

The symptoms of *Trichomonas* can sometimes be confused with thrush. The vagina and vulva become swollen and sore, and there may be tiny red spots on the inner walls of the vagina and cervix. Women with *Trichomonas* will usually notice a thin and foamy discharge, which may be white or greenish-yellow in colour and be excessively smelly. If the urethra and bladder become infected, too, there will be a burning sensation when passing urine.

Both men and women suffer from *Trichomonas*, and it can be sexually transmitted—passed from partner to partner during sex. It can also be transferred by hand and so is not confined to heterosexual relationships. *Trichomonas* can survive for a few hours outside the body. Women can become infected from moist towels and flannels. Even lavatory seats may harbour the germs for a short while.

It is much easier to detect *Trichomonas* in women as the symptoms are more immediate. The bug can be identified in the urine, but the normal procedure carried out at health clinics is to use a 'wet mount'. Some of the vaginal discharge is placed on a glass slide with a saline solution where the *Trichomonads* can be seen swimming about with their whip-like tentacles.

Trichomonas is treated with Flagyl (metronidazole) tablets taken by mouth. 90 per cent of *Trichomonas* cases are cured in this way. Regular sexual partners must also be treated as they may be infected too. Abstain from sex during treatment to avoid reinfection. Where both partners are being treated simultaneously, they may be allowed to continue having sex if a condom is used.

Flagyl should be used with caution. It is a powerful antibiotic and can actually cause thrush. Women who know themselves to be susceptible to thrush should take appropriate medication concurrently with the Flagyl.

Flagyl also kills off white blood cells. It should not be taken by anyone with blood diseases, or diseases of the central nervous system. It should be taken with food, rather than on an empty stomach. Alcohol should be avoided by anyone taking a course of Flagyl.

Flagyl has some nasty side-effects as well, which include severe nausea, stomach cramps and constipation. Recent studies have shown that Flagyl caused cancer when high dosages were given for a lifetime in some animals. If you have to take more than one course of Flagyl, you should wait at least six weeks before beginning the second course, and the manufacturers of the drug, G. D. Searle, recommend a white blood cell count after treatment. Flagyl should never be taken during pregnancy or while breastfeeding, as it can be excreted in the breast milk.

The use of Flagyl alone may not be enough to cure and prevent attacks of *Trichomonas*. Alternative treatments include using chaparral (see Chapter 6) and/or garlic and vinegar remedies. Like thrush, *Trichomonas* prefers less acidic conditions in the vagina and, again like thrush, can be prevented by controlling the pH balance in the genital area. *Trichomonads* prefer blood cells. An attack is likely to be worse during a period. Self-help remedies used around this time are particularly beneficial.

Non-specific vaginitis

Non-specific vaginitis is the name given to an irritated, inflamed or unhealthy vagina. Symptoms of this type of infection include an unusually heavy, white or yellow discharge. Sometimes this is streaked with blood. The vagina may be sore and itchy. There may be a burning sensation on passing urine, and other cystitis-like symptoms.

Although the germs causing the infection are unknown, this type of vaginitis indicates a disturbance of the finely balanced ecology of the vagina. The infection may be brought on by a course of antibiotics, or other drugs, as these tend to reduce the vagina's acidity. In more alkaline conditions bacteria and other organisms —normal inhabitants of the vagina and usually harmless there — rapidly multiply, giving rise to infections. Nylon underwear and tights, harsh soaps and/or vaginal deodorants can cause problems and provoke non-specific vaginitis. This is because these, too, interefere with the acid/alkaline balance of the sex organs. A vagina and vulva irritated from prolonged intercourse are also more susceptible to infection.

Non-specific vaginitis can occur when germs that live happily in *other* parts of the body, but *not* in the vagina, find their way here. The rectum, for instance, harbours a great many organisms, which can cause problems if they are introduced into the vagina or urethra. Both of these orifices are precariously near to the anus. By wiping towards the vagina, instead of away from it, bacteria from the bowel is easily spread around the vulva. E. coli, a natural inhabitant of the rectum, is one of the main causes of cystitis (see page 17). Urinary infections and non-specific vaginitis can be prevented by always wiping *away* from the urethra and by washing after passing a stool. Washing before and after sexual activity is also important.

Non-specific vaginitis can be treated. It is best to visit a special clinic where swabs will be taken to try to discover exactly which organism is causing the problem. If the infection is bacterial, a sulpha cream like Sultrin or Vagitrol will be prescribed. If no bacteria are found, the infection will probably be treated with tetracycline. It is advisable not to have intercourse during treatment and, possibly, to abstain for a short while afterwards, to allow the tissues to heal properly.

Non-specific infections can be remedied using the sort of self-help measures outlined in Chapter 6. These may also help to prevent recurrences. Garlic, with its antibiotic properties, can be effective in treating bacterial vaginitis. Insert a peeled clove into the vagina every morning for a week, removing the old clove before inserting a new one.

A non-specific infection may also respond to vinegar and salt water solutions. Doctors tend to recommend salt baths for women who suffer from vaginitis a lot, but, before you dash off to the bathroom, remember that frequent bathing can sometimes do more harm than good, and can possibly provoke an attack of thrush.

Gardnerella vaginalis

Gardnerella, or *Hemophilius*, is a strain of bacteria that has only recently been discovered as a cause of vaginitis. It is an infection of the vaginal secretions rather than of the vaginal walls, but, like most vaginitis, it occurs when the vagina's delicate flora is upset. Present in every healthy vagina, *Gardnerella* is only troublesome if conditions there become too alkaline. Like thrush, *Gardnerella* is very itchy. It produces a creamy white or grey vaginal discharge. This is often frothy, so it is not uncommon for doctors to mistake *Gardnerella* for *Trichomonas* or thrush.

The condition can be diagnosed at a special clinic. Unfortunately, the usual treatment available is a course of Flagyl (see page 73), which can trigger off an attack of thrush. Women with *Gardnerella* who are prone to fungal infections should always ask for a course of thrush treatment to take concurrently with the Flagyl.

Some clinics prefer to treat *Gardnerella* with sulpha creams and/or pessaries. Tetracycline is prescribed for the infected male partner. To prevent reinfection both partners *must* be treated.

A combined garlic and vinegar solution (see Chapter 6) may be used as an alternative treatment. Inserting *acidophilus* capsules into the vagina after each treatment with the solution to restore the vagina's natural acidity will help to prevent the condition recurring.

Chlamydia

Chlamydia trachomatis is a germ that infects the genitals and sometimes the eyes and throat. It is one of the most common causes of sexually transmitted diseases. Although it was recognized as an infection as early as 1909, it is only in the last 30 years or so that it has been taken seriously by doctors and health workers. It has to be diagnosed by specialists, so, if you think you might be suffering from *Chlamydia* arrange to visit a genito-urinary department of a hospital and ask for a test. Many cases are not picked up by tests at all, however, as the disease can lie in hiding for many years until it is triggered off by another genital infection or by a change of partner.

Chlamydia can cause cystitis-like symptoms when it infects the urethra and cervix — a thin vaginal discharge and/or lower abdominal pain, occasionally with fever. However, more worryingly, it may cause no symptoms at all. At least four out of ten cases of *Chlamydia* diagnosed in routine tests of women attending STD clinics show no symptoms at all. Meanwhile, the infection may have spread to the Fallopian tubes, causing pelvic inflammatory disease (PID), which can lead to ectopic pregnancy and infertility (three-quarters of the women who have three attacks or more are likely to become sterile).

Men can also by symptomless or experience a burning pain on passing urine and/or a discharge from their penis. In men, *Chlamydia* is often classified as non-specific urethritis (NSU) and may cause Reiters syndrome, a form of arthritis. Both partners should always be tested for *Chlamydia*.

In one American study, nearly one in ten of the pregnant women tested were found to have *Chlamydia*. It has been linked to miscarriage, ectopic pregnancy, and premature delivery. If the infection is left untreated, it may be transmitted to the baby during birth, giving it an eye or lung infection. If you are considering becoming pregnant, get yourself checked out for *Chlamydia* first!

Treatment is with tetracycline, an antibiotic, to be taken on an empty stomach. Pregnant women are usually given Erithromycin instead, and a newer drug, called azithromycin, taken in a single dose, is being tested for men with promising results. Like all sexually transmitted diseases, the best way to avoid it is to practise safer sex (see Chapter 9).

Atrophic vaginitis

This is not an infection in the truest sense of the word as it is not caused by a germ. It is often a plague on women's sexual health, however, and can be an indirect cause of thrush and other vaginal infections.

Atrophic vaginitis is an inflammation that occurs when the vaginal walls do not produce enough lubricating mucus. It is normally associated with the menopause, when the decrease in a woman's oestrogen level causes the walls of the vagina to lose much of their moisture and elasticity. The vagina then becomes more prone to infection. Intercourse may be painful, and the tender mucous membranes of the vagina are easily bruised and/or torn.

This condition can be treated with oestrogen creams applied directly to the vagina. A simple lubricating cream, like KY Jelly, which can be bought over the counter at chemists, will also help, particularly during intercourse.

Vaginismus

Like atrophic vaginitis, this is not an infection. Vaginismus is a medical term referring to a *spasm*, or contraction, of the muscles around the vagina, which makes intercourse difficult or impossible and very painful.

The cause of vaginismus may be a physical one. An unstretched hymen will make penetration difficult and painful. If penetration is attempted when a woman is insufficiently sexually aroused, the vagina may be too dry to accept her partner's penis. Perhaps, more important, are the emotional reasons that bring about vaginismus. The involuntary contraction of the vaginal muscles may be an unconscious protest against sex. Suffering with a vaginal infection such as thrush, even for a short while, can undermine a woman's confidence in her own body. One of the most distressing aspects of sexual ill health is that it makes the sufferer feel inhibited about making love. Learning to relax will help your vaginal muscles to relax and, thus, make sex less painful and more enjoyable. However, if you suspect that vaginismus may be caused by a physical reason, visit your doctor.

Non-infective leukorrhoea

Healthy organs and tissues are made up of millions of cells and the vagina, of course, is no exception. Throughout our lives, it is constantly replacing these cells — as old ones die, new ones are formed. The old dead cells are passed out of the body, unnoticed, with the usual vaginal secretions. The term 'non-infective leukorrhoea' refers to a heavy discharge that occurs when too many of these cells are being broken down. This discharge is usually white — so that it can be mistaken for thrush — and may be irritating. The increased amount of vaginal fluid may attract bacteria. Stale secretions around the vulva and in your pants will increase the likelihood of infection. Washing the genital area at least once a day with cool, plain water will minimize the irritation, but remember that a heavy vaginal discharge invariably signals a problem. It is always best to visit a doctor if the symptoms persist and/or the condition worsens. Non-infective leukorrhoea is more common in older women.

Cervicitis and cervical erosion

'Cervicitis' means an inflammation or infection on or around the cervix. Many women suffer from this complaint without knowing about it. They only find out after an internal examination or because they have another infection like thrush. Others experience a heavy discharge — white or yellow in colour, and possibly streaked with blood, or cystitis-like symptoms when the infection begins to affect the urethra.

The term 'cervical erosion' is ambiguous. Most doctors use the word as a blanket term to describe a red or inflamed patch on the cervix. Cervical *eversion* is frequently diagnosed as *erosion*.

The cervix is made up of two basic types of cells. The outer lining of the cervix is composed of pink cells, called *squamous cells*. Cervical eversion means that the soft red *columnar cells* from inside the cervix have spread on to the outer cervix, pushing the *squamous cells* aside.

The columnar cells arevery sensitive. They are highly susceptible to infection and can be brushed or damaged during intercourse. An *erosion* occurs when the cervix has actually been damaged and has lost some of its surface cells. It is rather like a graze. An *eroded* cervix looks red and sore because the delicate tissues normally protected by the squamous cells are exposed. Bleeding after sex, and/or bleeding between periods are signs of cervical erosion. An erosion/eversion or cervicitis may be aggravating a persistent or recurring thrush problem. For this reason, all three conditions need to be treated as soon as possible.

The medical profession still cannot agree whether *Chlamydia* causes cervicitis, or whether the cells of the cervix are just more susceptible to the infection when an erosion is present. However, it has been proved that more *Chlamydia* has been found in women with cervicitis than in those whose cervixes were normal. One study of women attending an STD clinic found that most of those who tested positive for *Chlamydia* also had some abnormality of the cervix, such as cervicitis or a cervical erosion.

Cervicitis is treated in much the same way as non-specific vaginitis — with sulpha creams or pessaries and/or antibiotics (such as tetracycline). An erosion or eversion can be successfully dealt with in one of two ways: by cauterizing the cervix, burning off the layer of cells, or with cryosurgery, where the cells are frozen. Some doctors prefer to leave an erosion alone, particularly if it is neither troublesome nor infected. However, if you continually suffer from infections like thrush or non-specific vaginitis, any disorder of the cervix must be seen to.

Cervical cancer

Cancer of the cervix is the most common of the cancers specific to women. Fortunately, it can be diagnosed at an early stage where the growth and spread of the cancer can be prevented.

Cervical cancer is detected by carrying out a smear test. This is simple and painless. The cervix is gently scraped with a wooden spatula. The cells from the the scraping are then examined under a microscope.

The results of the test will either be positive or negative. A positive smear does not mean that you have cancer. It simply shows that some of the cells are changing. The stages of cervical cancer are part of a continuum and the theory is that the changing cells can progress through the early stages to invasive cancer. This is still not fully understood because, even without treatment, the cell changes may stop at any stage, and even return to normal. Also, the speed at which the cancer develops varies greatly.

It is quite common for women to have abnormal smears. The majority of positive results indicate an infection or irritation of the cervix. An eversion would almost definitely result as a positive smear. Anyone with a positive result would be asked to return for a follow-up test, and for repeat smears every six or twelve months. Doctors in the UK are only paid to give cervical smears to women over 35, and to women who have had three or more children, but special clinics and family planning clinics carry out these tests as a matter of routine. Any heterosexually active woman should be screened at least once a year.

The exact reasons for cancer of the cervix developing are not known. Doctors think that there is a link between the cancer and sexual promiscuity, but how many sexual partners must a woman have before she can be labelled as promiscuous, and what about promiscuous men? It would seem that monogamous women whose partners frequently have extra-marital sex are exposed to the same level of risk as promiscuous women.

How can cervical cancer be avoided? Barrier methods of contraception may help — they are known to be good protection against VD. However, the most effective way of preventing cervical cancer is by making sure that regular smear tests are carried out throughout a woman's lifetime.

Herpes

Herpes are cold sores, which look like blisters or small bumps. They may appear on the thighs, in or near the anus, or on the buttocks. In women, herpes sores are typically found in and around the vagina, on the vulva and on the cervix. They are caused by the virus, *Herpes simplex 2*, similar to the type that produces cold sores or blisters around the mouth and nose. Herpes are nearly always transmitted sexually.

This is a most distressing complaint. The sores are normally extremely painful, especially if they rupture. Open sores are highly infectious, and they are, themselves, subject to infection from other bacteria. It may take anything from a week to one month for an attack to clear up. When the sores disappear, the virus enters a latent stage, when it is no longer contagious. A new attrack can occur at any time. There is no limit to the number of attacks a herpes sufferer may experience, although for many people the first attack is the worst.

As yet, there is no known cure for herpes. The symptoms can be relieved with sulpha creams and corticosteroids. Wearing loose cotton clothing and underwear during an attack helps. Try to keep the area cool and dry.

It has been suggested that there is a strong link between herpes and cancer of the cervix. For this reason, women who suffer from herpes should have frequent cervical smear tests, preferably every six to twelve months.

Warts

Genital warts, like ordinary warts, are caused by a virus, which may lie dormant for up to three months or more. They are infectious and are sexually transmitted, although they may be spread in other ways. They tend to grow more readily in warm and moist areas of the body. Women with a heavy vaginal discharge are more likely to develop warts, where they appear inside or outside the vagina or around the anus.

Warts can be felt as hard lumps, but they are rarely painful. In spite of this, anyone with warts should get them removed as they can be passed on to sexual partners.

Special clinics and doctors will treat warts. Small warts can be frozen off (cryosurgery). Usually, however, warts are burnt off with a weekly painting of podophyllum solution. The treatment must be continued until all the warts have disappeared. Any that are left will only spread again. As with all genital infections, sexual partners must be treated, too.

Crab lice

Intense itching around the genitals might be caused by crab lice, which infest the pubic hair. Like other types of lice, crabs are bloodsuckers. They attach themselves to the hair, close to the roots, where they bite into the skin. They quickly lay their eggs — or nits — which stick to the hair until they hatch several days later. This type of lice prefers coarse, wiry hair. They infest the pubic hair, but, occasionally, may be found in the hair on the chest, armpits, eyelashes and eyebrows.

Crab lice are usually transferred during intercourse, but they may be acquired through other kinds of close personal contact. It is possible to catch crabs by sleeping in the same bed as an infected person or from contaminated bedding and towels.

Normal soap does not affect lice. They are easily destroyed, however, with special shampoos, cream or powder, which can be bought from chemists or obtained free from a special clinic. Have a bath and dry yourself thoroughly before applying the lotion. Leave it on for 24 hours before washing it off. Away from the body, crabs die within a day, but the nits can survive for six days. Because of this, clothing, sheets and blankets should be boiled or dry cleaned or left for a week before they are used again.

AIDS

Strictly speaking, acquired immune deficiency syndrome, or AIDS as it is more commonly known is not really a genital infection, but it is spread through sexual contact. If, through unprotected sex with a new partner, you risk catching any of the other genital infections described in this chapter, then you also put yourself at risk of acquiring AIDS.

When this book was first written in 1984, few people in the world had heard about AIDS. Since then, AIDS has come to be recognized as a highly dangerous disease. There is now HIV infection in almost every country in the world, which, in turn, has brought about many other health problems. Medical opinion is divided about the cause and treatment of AIDS. Until we know more about this devastating disease, we must all take our part in stopping it spreading. The full extent of the AIDS epidemic is unlikely to be known for many years as the disease has now been shown to have an incubation period that can be in excess of ten years.

AIDS stands for acquired immune deficiency syndrome. AIDS sufferers have *acquired*, through the blood or secretions of an infected person, a *syndrome*, or group, of signs or symptoms that means that their bodies' defences against infections (their *immune systems*) do not work properly — it is *deficient*. Thus, AIDS prevents the body fighting infections in the normal way, so people with AIDS develop many different kinds of diseases that the body would usually fight off quite easily. Two common illnesses in AIDS sufferers are a type of pneumonia called *pneumonocystis carinii* and a form of skin cancer called *Kaposi's sarcoma*.

Most people think that AIDS is caused by the human immunodeficiency virus, or HIV. A person infected with HIV may feel well and appear healthy for many years, but, eventually, as the HIV destroys the body's defence system, a number of different health problems develop. These include fevers and night sweats, weight loss for no obvious reasons and exhaustion. Many people with AIDS develop chronic thrush, often in their mouths. Oral thrush is unusual in adults, unless they have just taken antibiotics or steroids, so an attack of thrush in the mouth should be seen as a warning that one's immune system is low. Research suggests that the onset of oral thrush in AIDS sufferers can be the sign that more serious symptoms will soon develop. Diet can play a big part in boosting the immune system and helping to ward off the serious illnesses associated with AIDS.

The HIV virus can infect anyone. This is how it can be caught:

- by having sexual intercourse or intimate sexual contact (such as oral sex) with someone who is infected (over 75 per cent of new cases are as a result of heterosexual contact)
- by injecting drugs with a needle or syringe that has already been used by someone who is infected
- by receiving a blood transfusion of infected blood (the chances of this happening in the UK are extremely remote as all donated blood is tested for HIV)
- HIV can also be passed on from an infected mother to her unborn child, or to her baby through her breast milk (all babies born to infected mothers are born with HIV antibodies, but many lose these antibodies as they get older, and, often, it is not possible to tell until a child is 18 months old whether or not they are infected).

The virus cannot be passed on through touching, shaking hands or hugging, therefore coming into normal contact with someone with HIV is perfectly safe. There are no reports of anyone becoming infected from kissing alone. Using a condom during sexual intercourse helps to prevent the virus being passed from one person to another, and practising safer sex will also help protect you from AIDS and other infections. You can read more about this in Chapter 9.

There is still a lot of fear and ignorance surrounding AIDS. Some people are scared to take an HIV test (a blood test that can detect antibodies to HIV), but, if you are at risk of getting HIV, it is vital to know if you are infected or not. If the result is positive, medical treatment can be started early, and you can make sure that you do not pass on the virus to anyone else. A negative test can be very reassuring and can help to ease anxiety. If you are worried about AIDS, speak to your doctor or call an AIDS counsellor. National AIDS helplines exist to answer people's worries (for the National AIDS helpline, see page 115; all calls are free and entirely confidential).

Hepatitis B

Like HIV, hepatitis B is usually transmitted through blood and semen, but it is more contagious as it can be transferred through saliva.

Hepatitis is a serious disease because it damages the liver, often irreversibly. A vaccine has been developed to beat this infection, but it makes sense to practise safer sex and avoid catching it in the first place.

Gonorrhoea

Gonorrhoea is an infection of the genito-urinary organs. It is only transmitted sexually — through intercourse or intimate contact with an infected person. This is because the bacterium that causes the disease — the *gonococcus* — cannot survive for any length of time away from the body. The *gonococcus* thrives in warm, moist environments. The organisms are transferred when natural moisture or discharge from an infectious person is deposited on the genitals of another sexual partner during intercourse. It is possible to develop gonorrhoea in the throat if oral/genital contact takes place. Occasionally sufferers may infect their own eyes.

Nowadays, gonorrhoea is far less common than it used to be, partly because of the increased use of condoms resulting from AIDS awareness. The incidence of gonorrhoea fell by almost 60 per cent between 1985 and 1988, and it still appears to be on the decline. Gonorrhoea, however, is still a very serious disease, because of the complications that arise if it is left untreated. It has also been found to occur in association with *Chlamydia*. So, all those who test positive for gonorrhoea should also be tested for *Chlamydia*, which, if present, will require different treatment.

Women with gonorrhoea rarely show any symptoms until its irreparable damage has been done. There may be a vaginal discharge and some discomfort on passing water, but, for most women, these symptoms are so mild as to be unnoticeable. In the majority of cases, women are not aware that they have gonorrhoea unless they are told by an infected male partner.

Except in very rare circumstances, men do develop symptoms, usually some two to five days after contracting gonorrhoea. At first, there is a burning sensation on passing urine. This is then followed by a penile discharge of yellow pus as the disease begins to affect the urethra. In women, the most common site of early, uncomplicated gonorrhoea is the cervix. There may be a cervical discharge. The urethra may also be affected. However, even in cases where both the urethra and cervix are involved, there may still be no warning signs of infection.

Sometimes small abscesses form around the external opening of the urethra. When the inflammation spreads along the urethra to the base of the bladder, it will cause cystitis-like symptoms. Sufferers will experience a frequent urge to urinate, although there may be only a small amount of water to pass. What little there is burns very badly.

Vaginal gonorrhoea may easily spread to the rectum as, in women, the vaginal and anal orifices are so close to one another. Infected discharge seeps into the anus, causing *proctitis*, or inflammation of the rectum. There may be few visible signs of anal–rectal gonorrhoea. However, some women do develop a slight anal discharge, more noticeable in the stools.

The early complications of gonorrhoea are severe, but they can be treated effectively. Without proper medical attention, however, the harm done to a woman's internal organs is often irremediable. The disease spreads up the cervical canal, through the uterus, to the Fallopian tubes — the tubes that 'carry' eggs from the ovaries to the womb. When the Fallopian tubes become inflamed, this is called *salpingitis*. You may have pain on one or both sides of the lower abdomen, accompanied by vomiting and/or fever. If the infection is allowed to progress further, the Fallopian tubes become twisted with scar tissue. This can result in complete sterility once the tubes become blocked.

Gonorrhoea must be treated at a VD or special clinic (see pages 35–37). These clinics offer the best facilities for the accurate diagnosis of all genital infections. Gonorrhoea is particularly difficult to detect in women. Discharge or a scraping from the cervix, rectum and urethra will be microscopically examined. Cultures of the *gonococcus* will be made in the laboratory. Sometimes a blood sample will be taken and tested for gonorrhoea.

Treatment is usually with a large dose of penicillin. This is given by injection, and ensures the greatest chance of cure in a large number of patients. When penicillin cannot be given — for example, when a patient is allergic to the drug — one of the tetracycline group of antibiotics will be prescribed. Patients will be asked not to have sex and to refrain from alcohol until they are completely free of infection.

Because gonorrhoea is so damaging for women, it is imperative to return for follow-up examinations. Repeated examinations and tests after treatment are essential as it is as difficult to establish whether the condition has been cured in women as it is to detect it in the first place. Remember that it is crucial to get prompt medical attention at the first signs of *any* vaginal infection (a vaginal discharge from gonorrhoea can easily be mistaken for other types of vaginitis), and if you think that you might have been exposed to the infection — even if you do not have any symptoms at all — go to a special clinic and ask for this to be checked.

9
Sex

> Although I am now thrush-free, I am an extremely frigid woman. I find it very difficult to make love with my husband although I force myself to and hope and pray that by forcing myself I will one day return to my former self, enjoying a perfectly natural and happy sexual relationship with my husband. I am also very sure that he suspects my frigidity — I certainly hope not — but how is it possible to hide one's true feelings from the one you love?

A permanent battle against a recurring vaginal infection devalues a woman's sexual worth, and her self-esteem. All too often when a problem affects our sex lives, sex itself becomes a problem, too. Thrush is irritating, painful and demoralizing, but the psychological effects it leaves behind, even if, and when, the infection finally resolves itself, are often the hardest to accept.

Sexual problems invariably inflict considerable pressure on any relationship and being unable to make love because of a scourge like thrush can be very frustrating indeed! Women who suffer a lot from vaginal infections need understanding and sympathetic lovers and husbands. Enormous amounts of patience and tolerance are required of both partners if the relationship is to survive the weeks of celibacy that make such heavy demands upon it.

Emotional stress complicates the problem. The lower you feel, the more vulnerable you are to the infection. It is another vicious circle.

> I have found sex to be the great aggravator and it all starts off again. Unless a course of pessaries is followed for about a month, then they don't work, and it's difficult to abstain for that long, or I start to get problems with the relationship, feel unfeminine and can't stand anyone near. It's an endless cycle of misery!

Thrush has serious repercussions in other ways. Women who suffer from vaginal infections may feel inhibited and lack confidence about making love, especially about oral/genital contact. Also, one or both partners in a sexual relationship may be unwilling to have intercourse for fear of provoking further attacks.

> At present, I honestly don't know whether I have thrush still or not. I am keeping my fingers crossed and hoping I can forget the fear of it returning since psychologically I feel the pain of intercourse, caused by thrush, has made me wary of resuming sexual relations.

It is sometimes difficult to decide whether or not a thrush problem is related to sex. For many women it seems to make little difference. Thrush makes its presence felt, month after month, sex or no sex. It is generally advisable, however, not to havee sex if you are feeling the slightest hint of vaginal discomfort. Tears and abrasions in the mucous membranes of the vaginal walls are an excellent breeding ground for bacteria that normally live (and die) without causing problems around a healthy vulva.

The chances of permanent relief from thrush rest on a good relationship between doctor and patient. Never allow a doctor to tell you to 'give up sex for a while'. Self-imposed celibacy is *not* a cure for thrush. Such comments are meaningless — how long is 'a while' anyway? Nor does it resolve thrush as it tends to imply that as soon as sex is resumed the problem will return.

Providing that an attack of thrush has cleared up properly, and that the tissues have been given time to heal, sexual intercourse should not be painful. It is quite normal to feel a little soreness after sex. However, an inflamed, swollen or itchy vulva would suggest that the condition has either recurred or has never been effectively cleared up.

> I used to dread having sex, because it would hurt so much and because I would invariably develop thrush afterwards. I was so tense that I could never enjoy lovemaking. I went to my doctor who said I was suffering from vaginismus and this was probably the cause of my thrush. Although my problem was an emotional one, it could be treated physically. The doctor told me that learning to relax the vaginal muscles is particularly important in preventing and curing vaginal infections. Exercising these muscles stimulates and increases the blood supply to the genitals. And when you increase the blood flow it means that more white blood cells reach the vagina to keep the area healthy.

During an attack

Never have intercourse during an attack of vaginal thrush as this will increase your discomfort. It may also prolong the infection. Thrush is sexually transmissible, too. It can be passed from partner to partner during sex. The chances of becoming reinfected are much higher if sex takes place again before the condition has been cleared. Men rarely show any signs of the infection, although they may be carrying thrush spores. Unless both partners are treated for thrush, it is likely that, as soon as sexual contact resumes, thrush will recur.

When both partners of a sexual relationship are being treated for thrush simultaneously, some doctors see no reason for lovemaking to cease. Bearing in mind how tender a vagina inflamed by *Candida* will be, though, it is sensible to forgo sex. Abstaining from sex for a short period of time allows the delicate tissues around the surface sex organs to heal themselves and will lessen the likelihood of the thrush returning. Do not be tempted, therefore! Do not have sexual intercourse while you are being treated for thrush. This may be some time, but it is better to wait than to carry on as normal, only to see the infection flare up time and time again.

Here are a few rules about sex that, if they are followed every time you make love, should help to prevent recurrences of thrush and similar types of vaginitis.

- Only have sex when it feels all right, and do not have sex during an attack of thrush, even if it is painless.
- It is good practice to wash before and after intercourse. This helps to wash away bacteria and prevent infection. Pouring cold water over the vulva and perineum after sex reduces any swelling or bruising that may have occurred during sex. This also helps to prevent urinary infections like cystitis because it washes germs away from the urethra.
- Go to the lavatory *immediately* after sex to flush away bacteria from the urethra. Again, this is particularly important in the prevention of cystitis.
- Until you are certain that an attack of thrush has been cleared up, avoid oral/genital sex. Remember that it is possible to develop thrush in the mouth.
- Many women are more prone to thrush at certain stages in their monthly cycle. Avoiding intercourse at such times reduces the

chances of another attack if the condition is aggravated by sex. For example, if thrush tends to recur just after a period, do not have sex during the period, and refrain for a few days afterwards until the 'danger time' has passed.

- Always use a sterile, water-soluble lubricant, such as KY Jelly during sex if you need to.

Thrush! Such an irritating problem in more ways than one. I've suffered with it for 11 years, since the birth of my first daughter. I found intercourse impossible while suffering and, of course, totally useless as it only made matters worse. I seem to start with thrush on most occasions when intercourse has occurred without good lubrication. So I make sure I've always got my KY Jelly at hand.

I suffered for three months with persistent thrush and throughout this time abstained from sex. The hardest thing of all for me was resuming sexual relations with my boyfriend. At each attempt I was incredibly tense and convinced that any touching of my genitals was going to be extremely painful, which made lovemaking impossible and the thought of penetration unbearable. This was such an ironical situation as, although I was thrush-free, I still could not make love.

However, through working in a hospital, I managed to see a gynaecologist. He showed nothing but kindness and understanding . . . and was very concerned that I should resume my happy sex life. He prescribed Aci-jel which, although it is quite messy, worked wonders because it supplied copious amounts of lubrication. The first time I was still apprehensive, but gradually I regained my confidence.

Safer sex

In recent years, the discovery of the HIV virus and AIDS has affected the public's attitude towards sex and relationships. The threat of AIDS is not going to go away — certainly not in the near future anyway, and possibly never. It is essential, therefore, to avoid the risk of catching the HIV virus. Practising safer sex will help protect you, not just from AIDS, but also from the other kinds of infections mentioned in Chapter 8.

What *is* safer sex? Safer sex is a term that has been coined as a result of people wanting to minimize the potential dangers of sex. *Unsafe sex* is:

- anal sex, which AIDS/HIV experts consider to be very risky, even with a condom.
- vaginal, anal or oral sex without a condom.

If you avoid doing these things, you will be practising safer sex.

The use of condoms has always been recognized as a way of stopping the spread of sexually transmitted diseases. Indeed, the British armed forces overseas have long been armed with condoms for this reason (they also use them over their gun barrels to stop water getting in, but that is another story!) It is probably true to say, though, that there used to be some stigma attached to buying and using condoms, but, more recently, condoms have been heavily promoted to the general public as a way of helping to prevent the HIV virus being passed from one person to another and so they have become much more acceptable. Using a condom also still radically reduces the risk of contracting other sexually transmitted diseases or passing a recurrent problem like thrush backwards and forwards between partners. This means that safer sex makes extra sense for thrush sufferers.

Condoms and spermicides

Since the spread of AIDS awareness, condoms are now generally considered to be part of everyday life. The condom is now the most popular method of contraception in the UK, couples seeming to have forsaken the Pill in its favour. There is now a huge variety of condoms available, even different colours and flavours. You can buy them from chemists, record shops, supermarkets, pubs and by mail order. The good thing about condoms, as mentioned earlier, is that they help to protect you against all kinds of venereal diseases, not just AIDS. These include herpes, gonorrhoea, syphilis, *Chlamydia* and genital warts. Condoms also offer protection against cervical cancer.

Nonoxynol-9 (N-9) is an active ingredient in most spermicides. This also kills some of the organisms that can cause sexually transmitted diseases, including *Chlamydia*, gonorrhea, HIV and herpes. Using a condom lubricated with these spermicides therefore offers better protection still.

Some women, however, find that they get vaginitis and/or

thrush-like symptoms after using spermicides. This is because these powerful chemicals can irritate the mucous membranes of the vagina and vulva, and may also affect the delicate pH balance. If you suffer a reaction like this, try to avoid using spermicidal creams or foams. This may mean changing from the contraceptive sponge or cap if necessary. Ask your local family planning clinic for advice. If you think it might be the condoms themselves that are causing the problem, change to a non-spermicidally lubricated brand of condoms. Those who are allergic to latex rubber can buy Allergy (hypoallergenic) condoms of Fourex skins, made from an animal membrane. Fourex are manufactured by Schmid Laboratories (for their address, see page 115) and can be obtained via mail order in most countries. Beware, though, they are not regarded as being as safe as latex condoms as a means of preventing diseases.

Female condoms, which line and protect a woman's vagina and cervix, are fairly new on the market. Research shows them to be as effective as the male condom, but they are not recommended if you have thrush or another vaginal infection. Also, if you are using pessaries to treat a bout of thrush, do not rely on latex condoms as the oil base of the pessary can damage or split the latex.

On a final note, it must be stressed that having sex with different people means that you are more likely to catch thrush or another kind of infection. If you do have more than one partner, it is a good idea to have a check-up every three months, even if you think you are all right.

10

Pregnancy and babies

> I got thrush for the first time when I was pregnant. In fact, I got all the symptoms of thrush just days after my baby was conceived. I'd never had it before and I hadn't a clue what it could be. I was so itchy!

> I suffered quite a bit from thrush when I was pregnant. It wasn't itchy, I just had a lot of discharge. I think this must have irritated my urethra as I used to feel a sort of burning sensation. It definitely wasn't cystitis causing this as the pain seemed to clear for a while after passing water. My consultant advised me on some self-help tips which worked well. Both the thrush and the cystitis-like feeling have disappeared now.

Many pregnant women develop thrush, even those who have never had an attack before. This is because, during this special time in a woman's life, her hormones change. There is more oestrogen in her bloodstream and this makes her body produce more mucus. Many pregnant women will not only notice an increase in their vaginal secretions, but suffer from blocked noses, too! These occur when the linings of the mucous membranes swell due to an increased amount of fluid there.

Thrush affects pregnant women because of the increased amount of glycogen or sugar present in their vaginal mucus. When too much glycogen is produced it cannot be broken down so quickly into an acidic form. This means that the vagina loses its natural protection against fungal infections. These conditions make a pregnant woman more susceptible to thrush.

Some women find that once the pregnancy is over, their thrush disappears. However, this may not be true in every case, and, anyway, nine months is a very long time to simply wait to see if the thrush disappears of its own accord. Also, the baby can pick up the infection during birth (see below) and, although this is easily treated, it is preferable for the infection to be cleared up before the baby is due.

If you are pregnant and suffering from thrush, tell your doctor, or whoever is supervising your pregnancy. Never use up the pessaries you may have at home left over from a previous thrush attack without asking a doctor's advice first. This is very important because there are certain drugs that should not be taken by pregnant women. Ecostatin, for example, should only be used with the utmost caution in the first three months of pregnancy. If you are in doubt about anything, always go and talk things over with your doctor.

Self-help in pregnancy

Pregnancy is the ideal time to take a gentle, holistic approach to treating thrush. Many natural remedies were detailed in Chapter 6, but it is worth mentioning a few of these again here. When used appropriately, natural therapies have no dangerous or unpleasant side-effects and are safe for use in pregnancy. They are effective against *Candida* and provide an alternative to drugs, which are best avoided at this important time.

Tea tree oil

Tea tree oil is *the* essential oil for expectant or nursing mothers. It is unique because it has both antifungal and antibacterial properties. Aromatherapists recommend mixing a few drops of tea tree with lemon oil in a burner to purify and scent the delivery room.

It is perfectly safe to use tea tree oil in the bath when you are pregnant. Mix a few drops of pure tea tree oil with about a teaspoon of gin (the alcohol dissolves the oil and allows it to be dispersed more evenly in your bathwater). Many pregnant women find this very relaxing and an effective cure for thrush.

Lavender oil

Lavender oil is another essential oil that new mums should keep a good stock of. Babies love a lavender oil massage. Add one drop to 100 ml (3½ fl oz) of almond oil and gently massage your baby after every bath. A drop of lavender oil may also be used to soothe a baby to sleep. Use one drop on the baby's cot sheet or clothing.

Bircarbonate of soda

Bicarbonate of soda offers another safe cure for thrush. Add a little to your bathwater or try the natural tampons treatment. Dissolve one teaspoon of bicarbonate of soda in a glass of warm water. Then soak a small, natural sponge in this solution and insert it into the vagina. Remove the sponge after a few hours and repeat several times a day or as often as necessary. If you do not notice an improvement after a few days, then it probably is not working for you.

Diet

Pregnant women should take special care with their diet. Women often use junk foods to ease their morning sickness, but sugary, refined foods make thrush much worse and might even bring on an attack, so avoid biscuits, cakes and sweets at all costs.

Concentrate instead on eating fresh fruits and vegetables. These will supply the vitamins that your baby needs to grow healthily. For example, iron and folic acid are necessary for the baby's developing nervous system. Eating leafy green vegetables, like spinach and broccoli, supplies you with these vital vitamins, but will not leave you constipated as a bottle of iron tablets often can. A nutritious, balanced diet will give you added strength and energy during pregnancy. It will also stop you piling on the weight, which means that you will have less difficulty regaining your figure after the birth!

Homeopathy

Homeopathic treatment is completely safe for expectant and/or nursing mothers, tiny babies and children as it has no unwanted side-effects. It can help relieve many of the problems associated with pregnancy, such as morning sickness, anaemia and water retention. Also, babies and young children respond excellently to homeopathic medicine because their systems are so pure.

Borax is one of the most commonly prescribed treatments for thrush. This can be bought at homeopathic chemists, but it is always advisable to consult a professional homeopath before using homeopathic medicines as there are many possible remedies for every illness. The homeopath's skill lies in assessing which one is right for *you*.

> Daisy had thrush — a sort of spotty nappy rash — which wasn't responding to the treatment my doctor prescribed. I consulted a homeopath who gave me one borax 30 tablet. A few hours later, Daisy's thrush seemed worse than ever — but this was just part of the homeopathic healing process. Her body was throwing the disease out of her system. A couple of days later, the rash had completely disappeared.

Babies and thrush

Young babies sometimes develop thrush in their mouths. This can be quite upsetting for new mothers. Fortunately, it is likely to worry the mother more than it bothers the child.

As mentioned above, newborn babies can develop thrush at birth. They pick up the infection from their mother's vagina during delivery. However, because babies' mouths are so warm and wet, it is quite common for them to develop thrush later on, too. Doctors will usually prescribe a yellow solution called Nystatin suspension for oral thrush. One dropperful must be squirted inside the baby's mouth several times a day. It may take a few weeks for this treatment to work, but it is absolutely essential to continue the medication for at least two weeks after the thrush seems to have disappeared. If you do not, it is likely that the thrush will come back.

> I was breastfeeding my baby when I noticed milk in the corners of her mouth. It wasn't until I tried to wipe these away that I realized they were patches of thrush. My doctor prescribed me some Nystatin suspension, I had to give my daughter one dropperful after a feed. I was told to allow at least an hour to pass before another feed to give the treatment a good chance of working. This was really difficult as she liked to be on the breast all the time.

Breastfeeding mums must also use an antifungal cream if their baby develops thrush. Nursing mothers can develop thrush on their nipples. This not only makes breastfeeding difficult, but there is a strong chance that the thrush will ping pong back and forth between a mother and her baby unless both are treated at the same time.

> When my baby had thrush in his mouth, I had to use Canesten cream on my nipples. They had become infected with thrush, too. They were sore and breastfeeding became painful. My midwife told me to spend as much time as possible topless to let fresh air get to them!

Smear a little antifungal cream on your nipples after each feed. Allow the cream to dry, but remember to wipe your nipples with damp cotton wool to remove traces of the cream just before your baby's next feed. Cool fresh air destroys thrush, so try to leave your breasts uncovered after each feed, and only wear nursing bras made from 100 per cent cotton. These allow your skin to breathe and will help prevent thrush taking a hold.

Nappy rash

Nearly all babies suffer from nappy rash at some point. It is thought that, at any given time, about one in three babies have it — some mildly and others more severely. Nappy rash first appears as spotty, red patches around the baby's bottom and genitals. It occurs when their delicate skin becomes irritated by urine or stools, or, perhaps, soap and detergent that has not been thoroughly rinsed out of terry nappies.

Nappy rash is made much worse if it becomes infected by thrush. Like adults, a healthy baby's body will naturally harbour *Candida* spores. Thrush will be present in a baby's bowel without causing any problems, but, when yeast cells in a baby's stool are left in contact with an area of nappy rash, the rash may become infected. Avoid nappy rash by changing your child's nappy as often as possible — thrush thrives in a damp nappy because of the warm and moist conditions.

If your baby develops nappy rash, ask your GP or your health visitor for advice. They will probably tell you to cover the sore area with a barrier cream until the skin heals. If they suspect thrush, you will be given an antifungal cream, such as Canesten or Daktarin. Smear a small amount of this around the nappy area and leave it to dry. Then, cover the infected area with a barrier cream. If the rash does not heal within a couple of days, go back and see your doctor.

> All the babycare books I read claimed there wasn't a link between nappy rash and my baby's teething, but the only times she suffered badly from nappy rash were the days just before her first four teeth appeared.

> My baby had nappy rash a few times and the doctor told me it was thrush. I used to put Canesten cream around his bottom and groin, then a barrier cream. It soon cleared up.

Nappy rash and thrush usually collect in the skin's creases. So make sure you carefully wash and dry these areas at each nappy change. Baby wipes will sting inflamed and sore skin. It's much cheaper and safer to clean your baby's bottom with cotton wool and plain, warm water. Make your own 'travel wipes' by soaking cotton wool balls or pads in warm water. Keep them in a small airtight plastic container, which you can easily carry around with you.

Let your baby spend as much time as possible without a nappy on. Lay your baby on a large towel in a warm room and watch the kicks of delight! Fresh air is a great cure for thrush.

If you use terry nappies, use one-way nappy liners as these help draw moisture away from the baby's skin. Better still, use disposable nappies until the rash has cleared. Avoid plastic pants whenever possible as these create extra warmth, and make sure you rinse towelling nappies thoroughly as traces of detergent and biological powders can aggravate a rash. Sterilize terry nappies frequently. Use a sterilizing solution or make your own by adding two tablespoons of vinegar to 4.5 litres (1 gallon) of water.

If you think your baby has nappy rash, you should act quickly to treat it. If you do not, it will quickly become much worse and, naturally, make your baby unhappy.

11
A way of life

Many doctors are becoming aware of self-help and preventative measures as treatments for thrush. In the past, women have often had to resign themselves to a lifetime of vaginal discomfort, celibacy and extreme misery. Today, learning to live with thrush is absurd. Learning to prevent it makes sense!

Out of sight, out of mind

Getting to know your vagina is the best way to prevent vaginal infections and to protect yourself against thrush. Few of us bother to examine our bodies very often, though the importance of regular self-examination cannot be stressed too strongly. Because our sexual organs are safely concealed between our legs they generally tend to be ignored. Surprisingly enough, it is possible for any woman to get a glimpse of her vagina and cervix, though she will rarely be advised to do so.

It is important to look at the external genitals so that the warning signs of a vaginal infection can be detected at the earliest opportunity. Most vaginal infections begin high up in the vaginal canal. By the time they hit the surface sex organs and become symptomatic, preventative medicine will have little or no effect. It is wise, therefore, to include internal examinations as part of your self-help programme. Doing so will help you to spot vaginal irritations, like thrush, before they become a big problem.

A do-it-yourself internal examination

Before you begin, you will need a speculum. This is a device used by doctors to separate the walls of the vagina so that they can get a clear view of the membranes lining the vagina and cervix. You can buy a plastic speculum from a surgical appliance shop, or ask for one at a special clinic or at a family planning clinic.

You will also need a mirror and a strong light. Use a directional lamp or a powerful torch. A non-greasy, water-soluble lubricant such as KY Jelly will help you to insert the speculum more easily.

Lie down on a sofa or on the floor. Make sure that you are

comfortable. Use a couple of pillows or cushions to support your head and shoulders. Insert the speculum sideways into the vagina, pushing it downwards and slightly backwards towards the small of your back. When it is fully in, turn the speculum so that the handles are pointing upwards. Slowly squeeze the handles together. This opens the bills of the speculum and holds the vaginal walls apart. You do not usually have to open a speculum as wide as it will go. The second or third notch along the ratchet should be wide enough. It is a good idea to practise opening and closing the speculum before you put it inside you.

Direct the light at the mirror and you will be able to see into the dark passage — your vagina. The vaginal walls will look very much like the lining of your throat. At the end of the vagina is the cervix, the base or neck of the uterus. You will notice a dimple in the cervix. This is called the os. It is the actual opening of the cervix into the womb, through which the menstrual flow passes.

You may have to adjust or reposition the speculum before your cervix comes into view. Its exact location will probably vary each time you examine yourself as, throughout the menstrual cycle, the uterus changes its position. The cervix lowers slightly just before menstruation.

If you have never done an internal examination before, you may want to get a friend to help you. The vagina may reject the speculum at first so reinsert it carefully, using more KY Jelly, until it feels comfortable. Never close a speculum while it is still inside the vagina. If you do, the bills of the speculum may pinch or nick the skin —remove it in the open position. Wash the speculum after use in soap and water. The plastic speculums that you can buy are marked 'disposable' but, as long as they are kept clean, they can be used again and again. It is best to sterilize a speculum if you use it during a yeast infection, but do not boil a plastic speculum — it will melt!

What you will see

The walls of the vagina are usually palish pink. If they appear to be puffy or red, this is a sign of inflammation and should not be ignored. A heavy white discharge indicates some sort of vaginal infection —probably, but not always, *Candida*. If the vaginal walls are white, it is very likely that you have got thrush. The white fungus might also collect around the external labia and in the folds of the clitoris.

It is normal to have a slight discharge. The membranes that line the vagina and the glands of the cervix secrete moisture and mucus. This moisture is usually transparent or milky-white and slippery. The amount and consistency of this discharge will vary throughout the month. For most women, is is slightly heavier at ovulation (about the middle of the menstrual cycle) or before a period. The secretions from the vagina increase when we are sexually aroused and during pregnancy. Also, the amount of vaginal secretion will depend on a woman's personal hormone balance.

Have a good look at the vulva, too. The outer lips, or labia majora, are soft and thick. They may be covered with pubic hair. The inner lips or labia minora protect the vaginal and urethral openings. The labia will vary in colour, from pale pink to dark brown. When we are sexually aroused, they swell and turn darker. Generally speaking, in its normal, unexcited state, a vibrant red, swollen or inflamed vulva is an indication of a vaginal infection, and it will probably feel as sore as it looks.

These broad guidelines should not be read as hard and fast rules. Remember that what is normal varies just as much as one woman's body varies from another. The best way to know what is normal for you is to keep a check on the vagina. This way you will easily be able to detect any abnormality. Keep a note of what you look and feel like when you do not have thrush, as well as when you do have it. You may forget what your vagina and vulva should feel like in their normal state, particularly after you have been suffering from thrush for a long time. Do not put up with vaginal discomfort. Remember that it is not normal to be in pain. A normal vaginal discharge is not offensive. It should not itch or sting. Never assume that an unnatural discharge or irritation indicates yet another attack of thrush as they could be symptoms of a very different type of infection.

Soreness or dryness, a strong smelling, dark-coloured or frothy discharge, itching or burning, or sore spots on or around the genitals are warning signs of possible infection. Symptoms like these could indicate a multitude of complaints. If you are in doubt, visit your doctor.

After a while, you should be able to spot an attack of thrush before it has properly begun. How often should you examine yourself? At first, inspect yourself every day — if this is possible. In this way, you will familiarize yourself with the numerous changes that occur throughout the menstrual cycle and you will build up a clear picture of what is normal for you at each stage.

Thereafter, examine yourself regularly — every week or so, for example, and at once if you notice an itch or twinge in the genital area. Conscious care of the vagina and vulva is your safeguard against disease.

Self-protection against thrush

It is a good idea to practise the following simple preventative measures and to keep to them at all times, as far as this is possible. Some of these have been discussed in Chapters 2 and 3, but they are mentioned again here because they are so very important if you are to keep thrush at bay.

Keeping cool

Thrush is exacerbated by warmth. This is why thrush sufferers generally experience their worst attacks during the summer, and why the itching and discomfort associated with the condition are likely to be more severe at night when you are tucked up in a warm bed. Making sure that the vulva is cool and well-ventilated will help to prevent thrush.

The weave of nylon and synthetic fabrics is impervious to normal circulating air as it is too closely knit to allow fresh air to pass through it. Nylon pants retain heat from the body. They will not absorb the natural daily secretions from the vagina. This discharge will collect around the vulva and, in no time at all, the crotch can become a very hot and sticky place. Such humid conditions provide an ideal breeding ground for thrush. Fresh, cold air destroys fungus spores; nylon pants encourage their growth. Always make sure that you wear only undies made from 100 per cent cotton. Change your underwear every day. Wearing no pants at all is a good idea, especially when you are recovering from a vaginal infection.

If you live in jeans then it is time to change your wardrobe! Tight trousers are actually a health hazard as they can cause thrush, and they certainly will not make an existing attack any better. They may also be responsible for recurrent thrush. Heavy denim jeans rub together when you walk, which causes friction. Friction generates heat, and heat, of course, means trouble. Wear loose-fitting cotton trousers instead. Providing that they are comfortable — to walk and sit around in — they should not cause you any problems.

I control my attacks by never wearing slacks, tight panties and

> anything made with man-made fibres. My tights have been converted into stockings with a pair of scissors. I have never connected attacks of *Candida* with either food or drink — only with heat and lack of ventilation between the legs, and man-made fibrous materials.

Do not wear tights if you suffer from thrush. Instead, wear stockings or suspender tights with an open gusset or one-legged 'tights'. The latter may be more comfortable than ordinary stockings. They are economical, too, as you do not have to throw both 'legs' away when only one of them is laddered.

Nylon trousers must also be avoided. Ski pants may be very trendy, but they are not conducive to good health. At work, many women have to wear nylon trousers as part of a uniform. Try to explain to your employer what happens when you are encased in layers of nylon all day long. Ask for a similar pair of cotton trousers to wear instead. It is just possible that the management are not aware of the effect nylon can have on a woman's body!

The craze for keep-fit continues and fashionable footless tights and leotards are a lethal combination to exercise in. Nylon and other synthetic fabrics are non-absorbent and impervious to air. After a session in the gym, the body is bound to become very sweaty. An attack of thrush can develop within minutes under such humid conditions.

> The main condition, I felt, that caused thrush to recur was when I got hot and sweaty, i.e. when playing sport — which I do a lot, or did, especially at school, and you discover that under your arms aren't the only places that get damp! I began to change my attire when doing strenuous sport or keep fit. I wore cotton running shorts and vests instead of these flashy nylon leotards and tights which thrush absolutely adores. I ensured that I had a shower straight after any exercises at sports halls or, failing that, as soon as I got home. A surprising number of people do not do this.

Hygiene

Keeping the genital area clean and fresh is the best protection against infection. Wash the vulva about once a day. This should be sufficient to keep the vagina healthy and odour-free, and will prevent the build-up of stale vaginal secretions. The easiest way to wash yourself is to pour cool, pure water over the vulva. You can do this squatting in the bath — using a shower attachment if you have one — or while you sit on the lavatory. Use a little plain soap around the anus. Part your legs and pour more water over the vulva and anus. Make sure that you rinse off all the soap. In very hot weather, pouring cold water over the surface sex organs will help to cool down a sweaty crotch and safeguard you against thrush.

Try to avoid baths and take showers instead. If you do not have a shower, crouching in the bath, pouring mugfuls of warm water over your body, will clean as effectively as any long hot soak and is kinder to your vagina. If you must have baths, bathe in shallow water. The temperature should be lukewarm or cool and try not to soak for more than a few minutes each time.

Baths are not very good for you, but they are far worse when you add strongly scented bath oils or foams to the water. Antiseptics and disinfectants are just as bad. Always make sure that the bath is clean before you put yourself into it! Traces of scouring powders and bath cleansers in the water can destroy the vaginal bacteria that help to ward off infections like thrush. Sitting in a bidet or a bowl of water is also quite dangerous. The water provides an ideal medium in which germs can work their way around the vulva and it is possible to wash thrush spores from the anus into the vagina.

Some women prefer to wash themselves with a flannel. This is a practice that should be avoided. Such cloths only harbour germs unless they are boiled each time they are used. Dirty flannels may be a constant source of reinfection for thrush sufferers.

Always wash your bottom after every bowel movement. Wipe yourself from front to back, wiping germs away from the vagina and urethral opening. Thrush is not the only germ that lurks in the bowel. E. coli is a natural inhabitant there and can cause endless misery when it finds its way into the urethra, as the hundreds of women suffering from cystitis will know. Toilet paper alone is not enough to stop destructive germs from spreading around the genitals. Thrush spores from the bowel must be washed away before they get on to your pants and work their way up to the vagina and urethra. If it is not possible to have a proper wash after passing a stool, wiping the anus with damp wads of toilet paper or tissues will suffice as an emergency measure. Pat yourself dry with more tissue or toilet paper.

Overwashing is also to be avoided, however, as this may disturb the natural biological defences of the vagina. Do not be too fastidious about hygiene and cleanliness. Remember that it is always possible to wash more germs *into* the vagina than you are actually washing *out*.

Washing your clothes

Washing should complement personal hygiene. Washing powder is a skin irritant. Biological detergents are more dangerous. The skin may develop an allergic reaction to the harsh chemicals they contain. The mucous membranes around the genitals are extremely sensitive. The way you wash your clothes can be significantly influential in preventing vaginal inflammation and infection.

Boiling underwear in plain water is the best way to wash your pants; there is no need to add soap. The high temperatures will destroy bacteria and fungus. Keep a special pan aside for this purpose. Alternatively, put your pants into a bowl or sink and pour boiling water over them. Leave to soak for about five minutes and then wash in the usual way.

During an attack of thrush, your underwear will have been contaminated by a lot of thrush spores, so that boiling is particularly important. To avoid reinfection, run a very hot iron over the gusset. This should remove any remaining traces of *Candida*.

Holidays

We all deserve a holiday every now and then. A change is as good as a rest — or so it is said. Even a short break can be a marvellous tonic. A chance to forget about thrush and really enjoy yourself! Ironically, holidays are often a nightmare for thrush sufferers. An abrupt change in climate and diet may spark off an attack, even if you have managed to keep thrush-free for quite some time. Suddenly, all the weeks of hard work, rigidly adhering to the 'dos' and 'don'ts' of a self-help routine, seem to be wasted.

Travelling for several hours in a hot and sweaty car or bus, stuck to a plastic seat, perspiring uncontrollably, is one of the quickest ways to develop an attack of thrush. This is because when you sit for long periods of time in the same position, air cannot circulate around the vulva. Stale sweat and vaginal moisture will begin to accumulate between your thighs. Add 'heat' to this moisture and you create an excellent environment for thrush. So, before you go on holiday, make sure that the clothes you intend to travel in are comfortable and loose. Do not travel in tights or tight trousers or you will be inviting trouble. At each stop along your journey, get out and walk about. Let some fresh air reach your perineum.

Thrush might start up on holiday, either if it is too hot and you have not taken suitable clothing with you or because of poor or limited washing facilities around you. It is pretty difficult to keep clean when you are camping on a desolate moor or hillside!

Another reason for getting attacks is that holidays by the sea tend to mean a lot of time is spent in water. Frequent dips in the sea or swimming pool are as bad for your body as long hot baths. In fact, swimming pools are much worse because of the chlorine added to the water. Chlorine is a powerful germ killer. It will destroy the *bacilli* that inhabit the vagina and leave it open to invading thrush spores. You can minimize the effects of chlorine by rinsing yourself with plain water after each dip in the pool. If it is possible, take a shower, but pouring pure water over the vulva will ensure that at least some of the chlorine is washed out of the vagina.

Change out of a damp bikini or swimming costume as soon as you can. Salt and sand will adhere to the damp material. They will chafe the tender skin around the surface sex organs. Pat yourself dry with a soft towel and use a little talcum powder around the tops of your legs if you are still a bit wet there. Always allow a swimming costume to dry out thoroughly between wearings, otherwise fungus spores might grow in the gusset.

On holiday, try not to relax the rules about sex. Wash before and after intercourse. Use lots of KY Jelly, too, or Aci-jel if you have some. These will help to keep the vagina sufficiently lubricated to prevent nicks in the vaginal walls, and will ward off vaginal infections. Aci-jel is especially good. It lets you have fun and maintains the vagina's acidity at the same time.

Do not be slack about your diet either. It may be difficult to say no to foreign food. Anything that you are served in a restaurant or buy from a take-away is liable to be high in calories and probably in carbohydrates as well. Foreign dishes can be very rich and spicy. They may provoke a full-scale attack of thrush.

On the Continent, the local wine will be flowing freely. Be careful if alcohol has been responsible for many thrush attacks in the past. Too much alcohol can also cause cystitis. Alcohol is a diuretic — that is, it excites the kidneys into producing urine. It is also a bladder irritant, so, if you are prone to urinary infections, alcohol can be more trouble than it is worth — a holiday with thrush and/or cystitis will not be much fun.

Try to drink lots of plain water during the day, especially if the weather is hot. Under a powerful sun, large quantities of the body's fluid will be lost through sweat. To prevent yourself from becoming dehydrated, drink plenty of non-alcoholic liquid. This will also help to negate the effects of a little alcohol in the evenings. Buy bottled water to drink, and to wash with, if the water on tap is at all suspect.

The best way to avoid thrush on holiday is to have a vaginal check-up before you go. You can do this yourself, using the self-examination method described at the beginning of this chapter. Alternatively, visit your local special clinic, Well Woman clinic or health centre. If the doctor cannot spot anything and you feel fine, you will probably be all right on holiday, but remember that an attack can strike at any time. It is better to take too many emergency supplies on holiday with you than to suffer in agony until you arrive home and can get treatment. The thrush sufferer's motto should always be 'be prepared!'

The following is a list of things to take with you in case of emergencies. It is only a basic guide and the amounts you will need will depend on the length of time you will be away.

- Canesten or Femeron cream and pessaries.
- Tea tree oil, cotton buds and/or tampons.
- KY Jelly or Aci-jel and some condoms, too, even if you think that there is only a remote chance that you will be needing them.
- pant liners, just in case you end up using the pessaries. They might not be necessary and/or you might be able to buy antifungal pessaries and creams while you are away, but it is better to be on the safe side and stock up with them before you go than find that you cannot get them and need them.

Keep remembering that, left untreated, mild thrush can quickly become quite severe. So, if an attack starts on holiday, treat it at once. Follow-up a course of pessaries with tea tree oil or any other sort of self-help remedies that you can get your hands on, such as yogurt- or vinegar-soaked tampons. This will help prevent further attacks.

If you prepare for the worst, there is no reason why an attack of thrush should ruin your holiday. Relax and enjoy yourself. If you are taking a hot, beach holiday you can enjoy the opportunity to wear as little (cotton) clothing as possible and let the air get to your body. Take the opportunity to go knickerless as often as you can because, as you now know, thrush hates fresh air!

Life-style

Looking after your body and your health plays an important role in self-help with thrush. Our hectic life-styles are very often detrimental to our well-being. Thrush is sometimes referred to as a 'nervous disease', which probably explains why some thrush sufferers are cruelly and mistakenly labelled as 'neurotic'. When we are feeling run down, or under considerable pressure, we have less resistance to invading organisms. Anxiety is a primary cause of psychological stress, and can be a cause of thrush.

Over-exertion drains us. Insufficient sleep, junk food and too much alcohol weaken our defences against infection. When we burn the candle at both ends, the body quickly begins to object. Keeping fit and staying healthy will improve the body's ability to fight disease, and exercise will increase the amount of stress that we are able to tolerate. Channelling nervous energy into any form of exercise provides an excellent outlet for anxiety and tension. Exercise will help both your body and your mind to relax. Exercise can be fun, too!

Getting rid of thrush can be very difficult. It may take time and it will certainly require a lot of effort. Like other fungal infections, thrush tends to recur. Treating the *symptoms* of thrush will not protect you against further attacks. The *causes* of the infection must be treated, too. Generally speaking, anyone who suffers from thrush will always be prone to disease, but with a better understanding of your body, by learning to recognize the causes of your particular thrush problem and learning to avoid them, thrush can be overcome. Even though there may be an occasional bout of thrush, your new awareness will help you to judge what you can do to treat yourself and what may need some medical help. In your battle against thrush, preventative care must become a way of life. So, keep at it — it will be worth it in the end!

Check-list

There are many reasons for our getting thrush. This check-list can be used as a quick reference guide to help you identify the cause(s) of your particular thrush problem. The notes in the right-hand columns suggest ways of avoiding further attacks — where they relate to a specific cause.

Possible causes	*Prevention*
Your health	
Recent illness? Antibiotics? Flagyl?	Avoid antibiotics whenever this is possible. If you do have to take antibiotics, ask your doctor for oral thrush tablets to take concurrently with them.
Run down? Not enough sleep?	Eat well, take plenty of exercise and rest.
Other vaginal infections?	Only thrush will respond to thrush treatment. Make sure you actually have thrush and/ or another infection. Get a proper diagnosis at an STD clinic.
Pregnant?	See your GP. Reread Chapter 10, use tea tree oil and bicarbonate of soda. Help cure thrush through your diet.
Diabetes?	Ask for a full glucose tolerance test. Vitamin B_6 tablets might help.
Menopause? Cervical erosion/eversion?	Ask for referral to a gynaecologist.

Contraception	
The Pill	Change brands. Try the progestogen-only Pill. Vitamin B_6 tablets or a short break from the Pill might help. Try another method of contraception.
IUD trouble?	Visit a family planning clinic for advice on alternative contraception.
Spermicides? Allergy?	Use non-spermicidally lubricated condoms and avoid spermicides altogether. Try Allergy condoms or visit a family planning clinic for advice on alternative contraception.
Sex	
Infection/reinfection from sexual partner	Always make sure that your sexual partner or partners are treated when you have thrush. Use condoms to prevent reinfection. Practise safer sex.
Alkaline semen	Use condoms. Aci-jel might help.
Prolonged/vigorous intercourse?	Use KY Jelly or other water-based lubricant.
Diet	
Poor eating habits? Junk food? Too many sweets? Sugary foods? Cheese? Mushrooms? Alcohol?	Reread Chapter 7. Follow the anti-*Candida* diet. Avoid sugary foods, white bread and other refined foods. Eat lots of live yogurt, vitamin A-, B- and C-rich foods and include plenty of roughage. Cut down on tea, coffee and alcohol. Try rotating diet to isolate 'suspect' foods. Avoid these foods in future.

Miscellaneous

Tights? Nylon pants?	Wear cotton pants and stockings, hold-ups or suspender (crotchless) tights instead.
Tight jeans?	Wear skirts instead of trousers.
Exercise in sportswear made of synthetic fibres? Nylon leotard?	Wear loose-fitting cotton clothes (shorts, skirts and so on).
Swimming? Long baths?	Always shower after swimming. Take showers instead of baths.
Vaginal deodorants/ deodorized tampons/towels/ ultra slim extra absorbent towels? Antiseptics in bathwater? Bubble baths? Overwashing?	Read Chapters 3 and 11 again.
Reinfection from flannels?	Boil flannels to sterilize them.
Reinfection from bowel? Systemic (total body) infection? Recurrent thrush?	Ask your GP to prescribe an oral drug for thrush. This may be the only way you will stop recurrent attacks of thrush. Follow dietary recommendations given in Chapter 7.

Oral thrush

Newborn baby affected?	Consult your GP or health visitor for advice. Carefully sterilize bottle teats, soothers/ dummies. Breastfeeding mothers should use antifungal cream to avoid reinfection.

In an adult? A course of antibiotics, anticancer drugs or steroids could be the cause.	Avoid antibiotics where possible. Ask your GP to prescribe an oral drug for thrush. Follow dietary recommendations given in Chapter 7.
Denture wearer?	Check fit of dentures. Sterilize dentures daily. Gargle with salt water.
Smoker?	Give up!
HIV positive? AIDS patient?	Consult doctor or specialist for advice.

On a final note . . .

Some women do not consult their doctor when they have thrush, they simply pop down to their local chemist for pessaries and treat themselves. Even so, doctors are now seeing more cases of *Candida* than ever before.

Sadly, it is likely that the incidence of thrush will continue to increase, for as long as doctors prescribe antibiotics of ever-increasing strengths, as long as the Pill is promoted as the preferred contraceptive over the condom, as long as women, persuaded by magazines and advertising, continue to buy vaginal deodorants and deodorized sanitary protection, as long as nylon and synthetic fibre underwear continues to be worn and as long as tights and tight trousers stay in fashion.

Drug companies have invested huge sums of money in seeking faster, more effective treatments for thrush, but it seems unlikely that scientists will ever come up with the ultimate cure that will make thrush a thing of the past. By following the advice set out in this book, however, it is possible to achieve such a cure for yourself. Self-help can control thrush and self-help will prevent reinfection. Even during pregnancy, when vaginal thrush can be so hard to shift, self-help will relieve attacks and reduce them to a minimum.

Much of the advice in this book ought to be common knowledge. If we were given more information on this subject, thrush would cease to be such a distressing and miserable complaint. In the past, women have had to find out about thrush the hard way. Now the simple solution is within easy reach.

Useful addresses

Homeopathy and herbalism

British Homeopathic Association
27a Devonshire Street
London W1N 1RJ

National Institute of Medical Herbalists
PO Box 3
Winchester
Hampshire SO22 6RB

Homeopathic medicines by mail order

Ainsworth's Pharmacy
38 New Cavendish Street
London W1M 7LH
Tel: 020-7935 5330

Gould & Son Limited
14 Crowndale Road
London NW1 1TT
Tel: 020-7388 4752

Helios Homeopathic Pharmacy
97 Camden Road
Tunbridge Wells
Kent TN1 2QR

Nelson & Co. Limited
73 Duke Street
London W1M 6BY
Tel: 020-7629 3118

Weleda UK Limited
Heanor Road
Ilkeston
Derbyshire DE7 8DR
Tel: 01602–309319

Information about chemicals and sanitary protection

Women's Environmental Network
4 Pinchin Street
London E1 1SA
Tel: 020-7481 9004

Washable sanitary towels

Ganmill Limited
38–40 Market Street
Bridgewater
Somerset TA6 3EP

Tea tree oil treatments

House of Mistry
15–17 Southend Road
Hampstead
London NW3 2PT
Tel: 020-7794 0848

AIDS

National AIDS helpline
0800 56723

Non-latex condoms

Schmid Laboratories
PO Box 2337
Anderson
South Carolina
USA

Further Reading

Carper, Jean, *The Food Pharmacy*. Simon and Schuster 1989.

Chaitow, Leon, *Candida Albicans: Could Yeast Be Your Problem?* Thorsons 1991.

Clayton, Caroline, *Coping with Cystitis*. Sheldon Press 1995.

Crook, William G., *The Yeast Connection: A Medical Breakthrough*. MD, Vintage Books 1986.

Diamond, Harvey and Marilyn, *Fit for Life*. Bantam Books 1987.

Gillespie, Dr Oscar, *Herpes: What to do when you have it.* Sheldon Press 1983.

Hay, Louise L. *You Can Heal Your Life*. Eden Grove Editions 1984.

Locke, Andrew, and Geddes, Nicola, *Women's Guide to Homeopathy*. Hamish Hamilton 1993.

Phillips, Angela, and Rakusen, Jill, eds, *The New Our Bodies, Ourselves: A health book for and by women*. Penguin 1989.

Tisserand, Maggie, *Aromatherapy for Women*. Thorsons 1990.

Weller, Stella, *Super Natural Immune Power*. Thorsons 1989.

Westcott, Patsy, *Alternative Health Care for Women: A women's guide to self-help treatment and alternative therapies*. Thorsons 1987.

Westcott, Patsy, *Pelvic Inflammatory Disease and Chlamydia*. Thorsons 1992.

Index